Independent CPhT Study Guide 2027-2028:

Prep Your Exam With 600 Updated Practice Questions with Expert Explanations and Rationales for Pharmacy Technician Certification

Yolanda Mensah

Author Introduction

The Certified Pharmacy Technician (CPhT) examination serves as a nationally recognized benchmark within the pharmacy profession, validating the knowledge and competencies required to support safe and effective medication distribution systems. Pharmacy technicians play an essential role in assisting pharmacists with prescription processing, medication preparation, regulatory compliance, inventory control, and patient support functions across retail, hospital, and specialty practice settings. The CPhT credential reflects a standardized level of professional readiness in medication safety, quality assurance, and pharmacy operations.

This study guide has been developed by an experienced examination content specialist with extensive expertise in pharmacy practice standards, medication safety principles, and competency-based assessment methodologies. The material is grounded in systematic analysis of publicly available examination content outlines and domain weightings to ensure structured alignment with the knowledge areas assessed on the CPhT examination. Core content areas addressed include pharmacology fundamentals, pharmacy law and regulations, medication order processing, sterile and non-sterile compounding principles, quality assurance procedures, and medication safety protocols.

The guide emphasizes applied reasoning and operational accuracy consistent with contemporary pharmacy practice expectations. Technical concepts are presented with clarity and precision to strengthen understanding of drug classifications, dosage calculations, controlled substance handling, insurance processing fundamentals, and patient communication standards. Rigorous editorial review and quality assurance processes were implemented to promote consistency, accuracy, and relevance to current professional pharmacy environments.

This publication is intended to serve as an independent educational resource for individuals preparing for the CPhT examination. Through disciplined domain mapping, structured content development, and adherence to professional competency standards, this guide supports comprehensive exam preparation while reinforcing the broader objective of advancing medication safety and professional excellence within pharmacy practice.

Table of Contents

Author Introduction **2**

Table of Contents **3**

Chapter 1: Role, Responsibilities, and General Duties of the Pharmacy Technician **7**

The Evolving Role of the Pharmacy Technician 7

Foundations of Professional Practice 7

Scope of Duties and Accountability 7

Communication and Collaboration in the Pharmacy Setting 8

Medication Safety and Error Prevention 8

Legal and Ethical Responsibilities 8

Public Health and Immunization Support 9

Technical Proficiency and Calculations 9

Quality Assurance and Continuous Improvement 9

Leadership, Professional Growth, and Advocacy 10

Scope of Practice and Legal Limitations 10

Medication Preparation and Dispensing Support 10

Customer Service and Communication Skills 11

Inventory Management and Medication Safety 11

Professionalism, Ethics, and Workplace Conduct 11

Chapter 2: Laws and Regulations **13**

The Legal Foundations of Pharmacy Practice 13

Regulatory Bodies and Their Jurisdiction 13

The Medicines Act and the Control of Medicinal Products 13

The Misuse of Drugs Act and Controlled Substance Management 14

Prescription Validity and Legal Requirements 14

Confidentiality, Data Protection, and Record Keeping 14

Liability, Negligence, and Professional Responsibility 14

Advertising, Labeling, and Sale Restrictions 15

The Interface of Law and Ethics in Pharmacy 15

Global and Institutional Influences on Pharmacy Law 15

Federal Pharmacy Laws and Regulatory Agencies 16

Controlled Substances Regulations and Compliance 16

Prescription Requirements and Recordkeeping Standards 17

Patient Privacy, Confidentiality, and HIPAA Compliance 17
Download Audio File and Flashcards 18
Chapter 3: Drugs and Drug Therapy 19
Principles of Pharmacology and Mechanisms of Action 19
Drug Classifications and Therapeutic Categories 19
Pharmacokinetics and Factors Affecting Drug Action 19
Routes and Forms of Drug Administration 20
Dosage Calculations and Accuracy in Therapy 20
Adverse Drug Reactions and Side Effect Management 20
Drug Interactions and Compatibility Considerations 21
Patient Education and Adherence to Therapy 21
Drug Storage, Stability, and Disposal 21
The Technician's Role in Therapeutic Optimization 21
Drug Classifications and Therapeutic Categories 22
Pharmacokinetics and Pharmacodynamics 22
Routes of Administration and Dosage Forms 23
Adverse Drug Reactions and Drug Interactions 23
Chapter 4: Dispensing Process 24
Prescription and Medication Order Intake 24
Data Entry and Verification Accuracy 24
Product Selection and Preparation 24
Compounding and Aseptic Technique 25
Labeling, Packaging, and Auxiliary Information 25
Pharmacist Verification and Quality Check 25
Dispensing and Patient Counseling Support 25
Inventory Control and Storage Management 26
Documentation, Record Retention, and Audit Readiness 26
Continuous Improvement in Dispensing Practice 26
Chapter 5: Medication and Patient Safety and Quality Assurance 28
Foundations of Medication Safety 28
The Culture of Safety in Pharmacy Practice 28
Identifying and Reporting Medication Errors 28
Root Cause Analysis and Preventive Strategies 29

High-Alert Medications and Risk Mitigation 29
Infection Control and Sterile Practices 29
Patient Safety and Communication Practices 29
Continuous Quality Improvement Programs 30
Risk Management and Regulatory Compliance 30
Ethical Dimensions of Patient Safety 30
Advancing Safety Through Education and Innovation 31
Chapter 6 – Practice Questions 32
Questions (1-100) 32
Answer keys and Explanations (1-100) 44
Questions (101-200) 57
Answer keys and Explanations (101-200) 69
Questions (201-300) 82
Answer keys and Explanations (201-300) 93
Questions (301-400) 105
Answer keys and Explanations (301-400) 116
Questions (401-500) 127
Answer keys and Explanations (401-500) 138
Questions (501-600) 149
Answer keys and Explanations (501-600) 160

Copyright

Disclaimer

Chapter 1: Role, Responsibilities, and General Duties of the Pharmacy Technician

The Evolving Role of the Pharmacy Technician

The pharmacy technician's role has transformed from a purely technical function into an integral part of the healthcare team. Once confined to counting tablets and labeling containers, the technician is now a certified professional contributing to medication safety, patient education, and public health initiatives. Within contemporary healthcare systems, technicians manage medication preparation, assist in immunization logistics, and ensure compliance with federal and institutional regulations. This expansion reflects the growing complexity of pharmacy operations and the reliance of pharmacists on skilled technical partners. The National Healthcareer Association emphasizes that certified technicians support both clinical and administrative functions that maintain the integrity of pharmaceutical services. They must demonstrate adaptability in diverse settings, from community pharmacies to hospitals, long-term care facilities, and specialty clinics. The evolving role also encompasses active participation in interdisciplinary communication and quality assurance processes. Through certification, training, and adherence to professional standards, the pharmacy technician has become an indispensable safeguard in medication delivery, ensuring accuracy, accountability, and efficiency across the continuum of care.

Foundations of Professional Practice

Professional practice in pharmacy is anchored in a framework of ethical responsibility, patient-centered care, and continuous improvement. According to the national model standards, every action performed by a technician must reflect a commitment to safety, respect, and competence. Foundational practice involves the integration of scientific understanding with ethical decision-making and compliance with legal requirements. A technician must recognize that professionalism extends beyond technical skill—it is a matter of public trust. Accuracy in dispensing, integrity in communication, and diligence in documentation represent the pillars of responsible practice. Continuous quality improvement is a defining expectation; each technician is accountable for identifying errors, participating in reviews, and adopting strategies that enhance patient outcomes. These foundations are not static principles but living commitments that evolve with advances in medicine, technology, and regulation. As healthcare shifts toward collaborative, team-based models, technicians contribute by ensuring that medications are prepared and delivered according to evidence-based standards and institutional policy. In doing so, they preserve both the scientific rigor and the ethical heart of pharmacy practice.

Scope of Duties and Accountability

A pharmacy technician's scope of duties encompasses all technical and procedural aspects of medication management under the supervision of a licensed pharmacist. This includes receiving prescriptions, verifying patient information, preparing medications, labeling, and managing inventory systems. Each task carries inherent accountability, as errors in these processes can directly affect patient safety. National standards emphasize that technicians must understand their professional boundaries—performing only those duties for which they are trained and certified—while recognizing when to escalate questions or discrepancies to the supervising pharmacist. Accountability is shared yet distinct: while pharmacists retain ultimate clinical authority, technicians hold personal responsibility for precision and adherence to protocol. Documentation serves as a record of this accountability, ensuring traceability in every transaction. The integration of automation and information technology further increases the technician's responsibility to maintain data accuracy and confidentiality. Whether working in retail, institutional, or compounding environments, the technician must exercise sound judgment and uphold consistent quality. This disciplined adherence to defined scope preserves public confidence and strengthens the operational backbone of pharmacy practice.

Communication and Collaboration in the Pharmacy Setting

Effective communication lies at the core of safe medication use. Pharmacy technicians function within a network of patients, pharmacists, nurses, physicians, and insurers, requiring both clarity and discretion. Collaborative practice depends on accurate transmission of information—dosage instructions, refill authorizations, patient counseling cues, and insurance claims must be conveyed precisely to avoid confusion or delay. Technicians are often the first point of contact for patients; therefore, they must communicate with empathy while maintaining professional boundaries. Active listening, verification of patient details, and respectful interaction form the basis of competent communication. Within the team, collaboration extends beyond task sharing to mutual accountability. Technicians must report potential errors, clarify ambiguous prescriptions, and contribute observations that support pharmacists' clinical decisions. Modern pharmacy environments rely on interprofessional synergy, where teamwork reduces risk and enhances care quality. Effective communication also extends to digital systems—accurate entry into electronic health records and adherence to privacy standards under HIPAA or equivalent regulations reflect both legal and ethical dimensions of professional communication.

Medication Safety and Error Prevention

Medication safety is a defining priority of pharmacy practice, and technicians play a central role in its execution. The Institute for Safe Medication Practices identifies recurring hazards—mislabeling, calculation errors, and look-alike or sound-alike drug confusions—as preventable through structured vigilance. Technicians must cultivate habits of double-checking, barcode verification, and clear labeling to minimize risks. Safety culture is reinforced through standardized procedures, incident reporting, and continuous education. A critical part of prevention lies in environmental organization: maintaining uncluttered workspaces, consistent storage systems, and controlled access to high-alert medications. Every technician's awareness contributes to the collective reliability of the pharmacy team. The ethical responsibility to report near misses and errors reflects maturity and professional integrity, not blame. In hospital settings, technicians also assist in sterile compounding and intravenous preparation, where adherence to aseptic techniques directly determines patient outcomes. By internalizing safety protocols, pharmacy technicians translate knowledge into everyday protection for patients and the profession alike.

Legal and Ethical Responsibilities

The pharmacy technician operates within a regulated environment that demands compliance with federal, state, and institutional laws. Legal responsibilities include maintaining accurate records, respecting controlled substance regulations, and following procedures for storage, labeling, and disposal. Ethical responsibilities extend further—ensuring confidentiality, honesty, and patient dignity. Legal frameworks such as the Controlled Substances Act, HIPAA, and CMS reimbursement policies intersect with daily practice, shaping how technicians handle prescriptions, insurance claims, and protected health information. Ethical conduct requires discretion, transparency, and the courage to address unsafe or unlawful behavior when encountered. Certification and continuing education reinforce awareness of these responsibilities. The relationship between law and ethics in pharmacy practice is complementary: laws define minimum standards, while ethics elevate practice toward moral accountability. Every technician must therefore balance compliance with compassion, recognizing that legality alone does not guarantee ethical care. Upholding both principles defines true professionalism and sustains the credibility of pharmacy as a trusted healthcare discipline.

Public Health and Immunization Support

Pharmacy technicians increasingly contribute to public health initiatives, extending their responsibilities beyond the dispensary to the community. Under pharmacist supervision, they may assist in immunization programs, patient education, and preventive care logistics. The Centers for Disease Control and Prevention's Global Immunization Strategic Framework underscores the importance of trained personnel in sustaining vaccine delivery systems. Technicians support this framework by ensuring vaccine integrity through proper storage, documentation, and scheduling coordination. In retail and institutional settings, they facilitate communication with patients about vaccination benefits and post-vaccination monitoring. The technician's role in immunization aligns with the profession's ethical obligation to promote population health. Through awareness of vaccine-preventable diseases and handling procedures, technicians bridge clinical operations with public health objectives. Their participation demonstrates how technical precision can have global impact—protecting individuals and communities from preventable illness while reinforcing the pharmacy's status as a frontline healthcare resource.

Technical Proficiency and Calculations

Mathematical accuracy is fundamental to safe pharmacy practice. The ability to perform precise dosage, concentration, and conversion calculations ensures that each preparation meets therapeutic intent without harm. Educational resources in pharmacy calculations teach technicians to interpret prescriptions, calculate flow rates, and compound solutions using dimensional analysis rather than rote memorization. This method fosters conceptual understanding and minimizes error under pressure. Competence in units of measure—metric, apothecary, and household systems—is essential, as technicians frequently translate between them. Equally important is the interpretation of percentages, ratio strengths, and reconstitution volumes. Errors in this area can have immediate clinical consequences. Therefore, proficiency in pharmaceutical mathematics is not merely academic; it is a moral and professional obligation. Through practice and verification, technicians develop confidence and precision that directly translate into patient safety. As technology advances, automated systems assist in calculations, yet human oversight remains indispensable—the technician's knowledge ensures that automation serves accuracy, not replaces it.

Quality Assurance and Continuous Improvement

Quality assurance represents the structured commitment to maintaining and improving the standards of pharmacy services. Every process, from prescription intake to final verification, is part of a continuous feedback loop aimed at error prevention and system enhancement. Technicians contribute by monitoring workflow consistency, identifying deviations, and implementing corrective measures under pharmacist guidance. The philosophy of continuous improvement aligns with professional standards that require reflection on performance and openness to innovation. Quality assurance is not reactive but proactive—it seeks to prevent errors before they occur through data analysis, training, and process evaluation. Regular audits, peer reviews, and adherence to documented policies serve as indicators of organizational reliability. Technicians, through routine diligence, help sustain these systems. Their participation in quality initiatives demonstrates professional maturity and reinforces public confidence. In a healthcare environment defined by complexity, quality assurance ensures that every medication dispensed carries the assurance of accuracy, safety, and ethical integrity.

Leadership, Professional Growth, and Advocacy

Leadership within pharmacy practice is not limited to managerial positions; it begins with individual initiative. Certified technicians demonstrate leadership through accountability, mentorship, and advocacy for safe and ethical practice. Professional growth occurs when technicians actively seek education, pursue specialization, and engage with evolving standards. This progression transforms competence into expertise. Advocacy extends beyond the workplace—supporting policies that enhance patient safety, access to care, and professional recognition. Within teams, leadership means modeling integrity, encouraging collaboration, and maintaining calm efficiency during challenges. The capacity to inspire trust and uphold standards reflects the technician's maturity as a healthcare professional. Continuous development also involves self-assessment and receptiveness to feedback, both critical for long-term advancement. By cultivating leadership qualities, pharmacy technicians elevate not only their individual practice but also the collective reputation of their profession. True leadership in pharmacy begins with ethical conviction and manifests through consistent, competent service to others.

Scope of Practice and Legal Limitations

The scope of practice for the pharmacy technician is defined by federal regulations, state pharmacy laws, and institutional policies that determine the tasks a technician may perform under pharmacist supervision. Pharmacy technicians play a vital supportive role in medication preparation and distribution, but they are not licensed to perform duties that require clinical judgment. Understanding legal limitations is essential to prevent unauthorized practice and ensure patient safety. Technicians may assist with data entry, medication preparation, labeling, inventory control, insurance processing, and customer service functions; however, final verification of prescriptions, patient counseling, and clinical decision-making remain the responsibility of the pharmacist. Scope of practice may vary by state, particularly regarding technician involvement in compounding sterile preparations, administering immunizations, or accepting verbal prescription orders. Adherence to established regulations protects both patients and healthcare professionals from harm and liability. Technicians must remain informed about updates in pharmacy law and institutional policy changes that may alter responsibilities. Working beyond authorized duties can result in disciplinary action, fines, or loss of certification. Effective communication with supervising pharmacists ensures that assigned tasks remain appropriate and compliant. By clearly understanding and respecting scope of practice boundaries, pharmacy technicians contribute to efficient workflow while maintaining legal and ethical standards within the pharmacy setting.

Medication Preparation and Dispensing Support

Medication preparation and dispensing support represent core responsibilities of the pharmacy technician. Under pharmacist supervision, technicians assist in processing prescriptions by accurately entering patient and medication information into pharmacy systems. Precision during data entry is critical to prevent medication errors that could compromise patient safety. Technicians retrieve medications from inventory, measure and count dosages, affix appropriate labels, and prepare prescriptions for pharmacist verification. In institutional settings, technicians may prepare medication carts, unit-dose packaging, or automated dispensing cabinet refills. Knowledge of dosage forms, storage requirements, and expiration dating is essential to ensure medication integrity. Technicians must follow standardized procedures when handling high-alert medications and controlled substances, maintaining accurate documentation to comply with regulatory requirements. Maintaining cleanliness and organization in the dispensing area reduces risk of contamination and error. While technicians support the dispensing process, final accuracy checks and patient counseling are performed by pharmacists. Careful attention to detail, adherence to workflow protocols, and strong organizational skills enhance efficiency and reduce risk. Through meticulous preparation and support activities, pharmacy technicians play an indispensable role in ensuring that medications are dispensed safely and accurately.

Customer Service and Communication Skills

Effective customer service and communication are essential competencies for pharmacy technicians, as they frequently serve as the first point of contact for patients and healthcare providers. Technicians must demonstrate professionalism, empathy, and respect while addressing patient inquiries, processing prescription requests, and managing concerns. Clear communication reduces misunderstandings related to medication availability, insurance coverage, or prescription status. Active listening allows technicians to gather accurate information and relay important details to pharmacists when clinical clarification is required. Confidentiality must be maintained at all times to protect patient privacy in accordance with healthcare regulations. In high-volume retail environments, technicians must balance efficiency with attentiveness, ensuring that each interaction is handled accurately and courteously. Communication extends beyond patient interaction and includes collaboration with pharmacists, prescribers, insurance representatives, and other healthcare professionals. Telephone etiquette and proper documentation of conversations are essential components of professional conduct. When faced with challenging situations, such as frustrated or distressed patients, technicians must remain calm and seek pharmacist involvement when appropriate. Strong communication skills foster trust, enhance patient satisfaction, and contribute to the overall effectiveness of pharmacy operations.

Inventory Management and Medication Safety

Inventory management is a critical responsibility that ensures medications are available, properly stored, and safe for patient use. Pharmacy technicians monitor stock levels, rotate inventory to prevent expiration, and verify deliveries against purchase orders. Proper storage conditions, including temperature control and protection from light or moisture, preserve medication potency and stability. Controlled substances require additional safeguards, including secure storage and meticulous recordkeeping to comply with federal regulations. Technicians assist with regular inventory audits and reconciliation to detect discrepancies or diversion. Removing expired or recalled products from stock protects patients from ineffective or harmful medications. Familiarity with medication safety practices reduces the likelihood of dispensing errors, particularly with look-alike or sound-alike drug names. Organized shelving and clear labeling enhance workflow efficiency and accuracy. Inventory control also involves anticipating demand patterns and coordinating timely reordering to prevent shortages. Through diligent oversight of medication storage and distribution processes, pharmacy technicians support patient safety and regulatory compliance within the pharmacy setting.

Professionalism, Ethics, and Workplace Conduct

Professionalism and ethical conduct are fundamental expectations for pharmacy technicians. Ethical practice includes honesty, integrity, accountability, and respect for patients and colleagues. Technicians must adhere to confidentiality standards and avoid conflicts of interest that could compromise patient trust. Maintaining professional boundaries and appropriate workplace behavior fosters a respectful and collaborative environment. Reliability and punctuality contribute to efficient workflow and demonstrate commitment to team responsibilities. Ethical dilemmas may arise when errors occur or when questionable practices are observed; technicians have a duty to report concerns to supervising pharmacists or appropriate authorities. Commitment to ethical standards strengthens public confidence in pharmacy services. Professional appearance and demeanor further reinforce credibility. Continuous self-improvement and receptiveness to feedback enhance competence and career growth. By embodying ethical principles and maintaining professional conduct, pharmacy technicians uphold the integrity of the pharmacy profession and support safe, patient-centered care.

Chapter 2: Laws and Regulations

The Legal Foundations of Pharmacy Practice

Pharmacy law establishes the structure through which medicines are controlled, dispensed, and monitored in the interest of public safety. It defines the pharmacist's and technician's obligations, delineates professional accountability, and ensures consistency across all healthcare settings. Central to this legal framework are statutes such as the Medicines Act, which governs the licensing and supply of medicinal products, and the Misuse of Drugs Act, which controls substances with potential for abuse. The technician's role exists within this statutory ecosystem, requiring compliance with both national legislation and institutional policy. Law in pharmacy is preventive rather than punitive; it aims to forestall harm by creating procedural safeguards. Documentation, verification, and traceability are all legal imperatives designed to ensure patient safety and uphold professional transparency. As healthcare advances, law evolves to address technological innovation, digital records, and patient privacy. Understanding these legal foundations allows technicians to act not as passive operators but as active guardians of ethical and lawful practice within the pharmacy environment.

Regulatory Bodies and Their Jurisdiction

Regulatory agencies provide the oversight that ensures public trust in the handling and supply of medicines. Institutions such as the national medicines regulatory authority, public health departments, and professional councils each hold defined jurisdictional authority. The pharmacy technician operates within this network, following the standards issued by these bodies to ensure safety, legality, and quality. For example, the regulation of controlled substances involves coordination between law enforcement, licensing boards, and pharmacy management. These agencies also govern the processes of registration, continuing education, and discipline. Their collective purpose is to harmonize practice with both statutory and ethical standards. When a breach occurs, these regulators initiate investigation and corrective measures, preserving the credibility of the profession. Compliance with their guidance is not optional—it is a condition of lawful practice. By maintaining awareness of current regulations, technicians contribute to a culture of integrity and protect the profession from reputational risk.

The Medicines Act and the Control of Medicinal Products

The Medicines Act provides the comprehensive framework for the manufacture, sale, and distribution of medicinal products. It distinguishes between prescription-only, pharmacy, and general sale medicines, ensuring that products are supplied through appropriate channels. The Act requires that all medicinal products possess proper authorization before being marketed, ensuring they meet standards of safety, efficacy, and quality. Pharmacy technicians must understand how these classifications affect dispensing responsibilities. A medicine without authorization may not be legally supplied except under specified exemptions, such as hospital use or named-patient supply. The Act also regulates labeling, storage, and record-keeping—areas directly managed by technicians. By adhering to these provisions, technicians prevent the circulation of counterfeit, substandard, or misbranded medicines. The law thus transforms ordinary tasks—checking expiry dates, maintaining temperature logs, or labeling containers—into legal obligations. This relationship between routine process and legislative compliance forms the foundation of lawful pharmaceutical service and reinforces the profession's accountability to the public.

The Misuse of Drugs Act and Controlled Substance Management

Controlled substances present unique legal challenges because of their potential for dependency, diversion, and misuse. The Misuse of Drugs Act and associated regulations provide strict controls over their classification, storage, prescription, and destruction. Pharmacy technicians play a direct role in ensuring compliance by maintaining accurate records, verifying authorization, and monitoring quantities. The law requires controlled drugs to be stored securely in locked cabinets and for all transactions to be recorded in permanent registers. Any discrepancies must be reported immediately to the supervising pharmacist or relevant authority. Mismanagement of controlled substances carries severe legal consequences, including criminal liability. However, beyond fear of penalty, these measures reinforce professional responsibility. The technician's vigilance ensures that potent medications reach only those who need them, in the correct form and dosage. Legal control of drugs under this Act exemplifies how technical precision intersects with ethical duty, safeguarding both patient welfare and the public interest.

Prescription Validity and Legal Requirements

A valid prescription is a legal document authorizing the preparation and supply of a medicinal product to a named individual. Laws governing prescriptions define mandatory elements such as patient identification, prescriber credentials, dosage instructions, and date of issue. Pharmacy technicians must recognize that the prescription is both a medical order and a legal instrument; any omission or ambiguity can render it invalid. Regulations also dictate the time frame for dispensing and the specific documentation required for controlled substances. Alteration, misuse, or unauthorized duplication of prescriptions constitutes a legal offense. Technicians are expected to identify irregularities and seek clarification from the pharmacist before proceeding. These safeguards are designed to prevent errors, forgery, and inappropriate therapy. By adhering to prescription law, the technician not only complies with regulation but also contributes to clinical accuracy and patient protection. Every filled prescription thus represents a lawful act grounded in both technical precision and professional judgment.

Confidentiality, Data Protection, and Record Keeping

Confidentiality in pharmacy practice is a legal and ethical cornerstone. Legislation on data protection mandates that personal health information be collected, stored, and disclosed only for legitimate healthcare purposes. Pharmacy technicians must ensure that records—whether electronic or paper—remain secure and accessible only to authorized personnel. Conversations regarding a patient's therapy must occur discreetly to prevent breaches of privacy. Laws governing confidentiality extend to prescription records, insurance claims, and communications with prescribers. Unauthorized disclosure can result in legal sanction and professional discipline. Record keeping serves dual functions: it maintains continuity of care and establishes evidence of compliance with law. Accurate documentation of dispensing, counseling, and incident reports demonstrates accountability. In an era of electronic health records, technicians must understand how digital privacy regulations interface with pharmacy systems. Upholding confidentiality is therefore not an isolated rule but a daily discipline reflecting the profession's respect for patient dignity and public trust.

Liability, Negligence, and Professional Responsibility

Liability law defines accountability when harm arises from professional action or omission. In pharmacy, negligence may occur through dispensing errors, failure to follow procedure, or inadequate supervision.

Even though technicians work under pharmacist oversight, they hold personal responsibility for tasks within their competence. Legal cases have established that both pharmacists and technicians share the duty of care owed to patients. To avoid negligence, technicians must adhere strictly to standard operating procedures and maintain competence through ongoing education. Errors are evaluated based on whether reasonable care was exercised, not on intent. Proper documentation and communication with the supervising pharmacist serve as the best defense against liability claims. The law recognizes human error but demands systematic prevention and prompt correction. Ultimately, professional responsibility is not only about avoiding legal consequences—it is about affirming the moral and legal commitment to patient safety that defines the profession's credibility.

Advertising, Labeling, and Sale Restrictions

Pharmaceutical advertising and labeling are subject to precise legal regulation to protect consumers from misleading claims and unsafe products. The law requires that all medicinal packaging contain accurate information about composition, dosage, contraindications, and storage. Pharmacy technicians are responsible for ensuring that labels generated in dispensing accurately reflect prescriber instructions and comply with legal standards for clarity and content. Mislabeling constitutes a serious breach that can lead to disciplinary or criminal action. Similarly, sale restrictions under the Medicines Act prohibit the unauthorized sale of prescription-only medications and govern over-the-counter classifications. Technicians must understand the distinctions between these categories to ensure lawful supply. Advertising of medicines to the public is limited by legislation that seeks to prevent self-diagnosis and misuse. In practice, adherence to labeling and sale regulations ensures not only compliance but also trust. Patients rely on pharmacies as regulated environments where accuracy and honesty are legal guarantees.

The Interface of Law and Ethics in Pharmacy

Law defines the boundaries of permissible conduct, while ethics guides the moral choices within those boundaries. Pharmacy technicians navigate both frameworks daily. While legal compliance ensures that actions meet statutory requirements, ethical reasoning determines whether those actions also reflect compassion and fairness. For instance, confidentiality may be legally mandated, but the ethical dimension requires empathy when handling sensitive information. The law provides structure, but ethics supplies conscience. Together, they sustain professionalism and social trust. Technicians must recognize that not every ethical dilemma is addressed explicitly in legislation; judgment, guided by training and professional codes, bridges the gap. When conflicts arise—between legal obligation and personal conviction—the appropriate course involves consultation and adherence to institutional policy. Mastery of both law and ethics allows technicians to serve with confidence and integrity, fulfilling their dual responsibility to the healthcare system and the communities they support.

Global and Institutional Influences on Pharmacy Law

Pharmacy law does not exist in isolation; it evolves within global and institutional contexts. International agreements, such as those governing drug control or trade standards, influence national legislation. Public health emergencies, emerging diseases, and technological innovations continually reshape the regulatory landscape. Within healthcare institutions, internal policies translate these broad laws into operational procedures that guide technicians' daily work. Hospitals, retail chains, and regulatory agencies interpret legal requirements through their own governance structures. Technicians must therefore remain alert to both statutory law and organizational policy, ensuring that practice remains current and compliant.

Globalization has also introduced new ethical and logistical challenges, including cross-border medication supply and counterfeit drug prevention. The intersection of local law with international principles reflects the profession's expanding scope and responsibility. Understanding these influences prepares pharmacy technicians to adapt to a dynamic legal environment while preserving the unwavering priority of patient safety.

Federal Pharmacy Laws and Regulatory Agencies

Federal pharmacy laws establish the legal framework governing medication distribution, controlled substances, drug approval, and patient safety across the United States. Pharmacy technicians must understand the role of major regulatory agencies, particularly the Food and Drug Administration and the Drug Enforcement Administration. The Food and Drug Administration is responsible for approving new medications, monitoring drug safety, regulating manufacturing standards, and overseeing labeling requirements. The Drug Enforcement Administration enforces laws related to controlled substances, including registration of pharmacies, prescribers, and wholesalers. The Controlled Substances Act categorizes drugs into schedules based on medical use, potential for abuse, and risk of dependence. Pharmacy technicians must recognize schedule classifications and understand storage, documentation, and dispensing restrictions for each category. Federal law also regulates prescription transfers, refills, record retention, and electronic prescribing standards. Technicians must comply with these requirements to prevent diversion and maintain legal operation of the pharmacy. Violations of federal pharmacy law can result in severe penalties, including fines, loss of licensure, or criminal charges. Staying informed about regulatory updates and maintaining accurate documentation ensures compliance. Knowledge of federal oversight supports safe medication practices and protects public health while reinforcing the pharmacy technician's legal responsibilities within the healthcare system.

Controlled Substances Regulations and Compliance

Controlled substances require heightened regulatory oversight due to their potential for abuse and diversion. Pharmacy technicians play an important role in maintaining compliance with federal and state regulations governing these medications. Controlled drugs are categorized into five schedules, with Schedule I substances having no accepted medical use and Schedule II through V medications having decreasing abuse potential. Schedule II medications have strict prescribing and refill limitations, while lower schedules allow varying degrees of refill authorization. Technicians must ensure secure storage of controlled substances in locked cabinets or designated areas with restricted access. Accurate recordkeeping is mandatory, including documentation of receipt, dispensing, transfers, and inventory counts. Pharmacies are required to conduct regular controlled substance inventories and reconcile discrepancies promptly. Prescription requirements differ by schedule, including written or electronic prescribing mandates and limitations on verbal orders. Technicians must verify completeness of prescriptions before processing and refer any irregularities to the pharmacist. Reporting of theft or significant loss to regulatory authorities is a legal obligation. Failure to adhere to controlled substance regulations may result in serious legal consequences for both the pharmacy and individual staff members. Strict compliance safeguards against diversion and supports responsible medication management practices.

Prescription Requirements and Recordkeeping Standards

Accurate prescription processing and proper recordkeeping are fundamental components of pharmacy law compliance. A valid prescription must include essential elements such as patient name, prescriber information, medication name, strength, dosage form, quantity, directions for use, and authorized refills. Technicians are responsible for verifying completeness of these components during data entry while deferring clinical evaluation to the pharmacist. Electronic prescribing systems must meet federal and state security standards to prevent fraud or unauthorized alterations. Record retention requirements vary depending on federal and state regulations but generally mandate preservation of prescription records, controlled substance logs, and inventory documentation for specified timeframes. Proper filing systems, whether electronic or paper-based, ensure accessibility during audits or inspections. Documentation must be clear, legible, and accurate to support traceability and legal accountability. Incomplete or inaccurate records can result in regulatory penalties or jeopardize patient safety. Confidentiality laws require secure storage of patient information and restricted access to authorized personnel. Technicians must also follow procedures for prescription transfers between pharmacies, ensuring compliance with applicable regulations. Thorough understanding of prescription requirements and meticulous recordkeeping practices promote operational integrity and protect both patients and pharmacy personnel.

Patient Privacy, Confidentiality, and HIPAA Compliance

Patient privacy and confidentiality are critical legal obligations within pharmacy practice. The Health Insurance Portability and Accountability Act establishes national standards for protecting individually identifiable health information. Pharmacy technicians routinely handle protected health information, including prescription details, medical conditions, insurance data, and personal identifiers. Compliance requires limiting access to authorized individuals and safeguarding both electronic and paper records. Conversations involving patient information must be conducted discreetly to prevent unauthorized disclosure. Computer systems should be secured with unique login credentials and automatic log-off features to reduce risk of breaches. Disclosure of protected health information without patient authorization is permitted only under specific circumstances defined by law, such as public health reporting or law enforcement requests. Violations of privacy regulations can result in substantial fines, legal consequences, and reputational harm to the pharmacy. Technicians must complete training on privacy standards and remain vigilant against potential data breaches or phishing attempts. Proper disposal of sensitive documents through shredding and secure electronic data management further protects confidentiality. Upholding privacy standards reinforces patient trust and ensures compliance with federal and state regulations governing healthcare information security.

Download Audio File and Flashcards

Chapter 3: Drugs and Drug Therapy

Principles of Pharmacology and Mechanisms of Action

Pharmacology is the scientific foundation upon which all aspects of drug therapy rest. It studies how chemical substances interact with living systems to produce therapeutic effects or adverse reactions. Every medication acts through a mechanism of action—an interaction between the drug and specific biological targets such as enzymes, receptors, or ion channels. These interactions determine the drug's efficacy and selectivity. Understanding pharmacodynamics (what the drug does to the body) and pharmacokinetics (what the body does to the drug) enables technicians to anticipate responses and recognize deviations from expected outcomes. Absorption, distribution, metabolism, and excretion—collectively known as ADME—govern drug behavior in the body. Variations in these processes explain differences in patient response, especially when influenced by age, genetics, or concurrent medications. For the pharmacy technician, knowledge of pharmacology ensures that medication preparation and counseling support the prescriber's intent. Each step, from verifying dosage forms to checking interactions, reflects a grasp of pharmacologic principles that safeguard the balance between efficacy and safety.

Drug Classifications and Therapeutic Categories

Medications are categorized according to their chemical properties, mechanisms, and therapeutic applications. Drug classification provides an organized framework for understanding how agents treat specific conditions. For example, antibiotics target bacterial infections through inhibition of cell wall synthesis or protein production, while antihypertensives lower blood pressure by dilating vessels or reducing cardiac workload. These classifications guide proper storage, labeling, and counseling in the pharmacy setting. Technicians must recognize common classes—analgesics, antivirals, antidiabetics, antidepressants, and others—to assist pharmacists in identifying potential contraindications or duplications in therapy. Classification also determines how a drug is scheduled or controlled under law. In practice, technicians rely on classification knowledge to interpret prescriptions accurately, locate appropriate stock, and avoid dispensing errors between look-alike or sound-alike medications. The systematic understanding of drug categories transforms what might appear as a list of names into an interrelated network of therapeutic strategies designed to restore or maintain health.

Pharmacokinetics and Factors Affecting Drug Action

Pharmacokinetics describes the movement of drugs within the body—how they are absorbed, distributed, metabolized, and eliminated. Absorption determines how quickly and effectively a drug enters the bloodstream, influenced by route of administration, solubility, and formulation. Distribution depends on blood flow, protein binding, and tissue permeability, determining where a drug exerts its effects. Metabolism, primarily in the liver, converts active substances into forms that can be excreted, while elimination through the kidneys or bile finalizes the process. Several patient-specific factors alter these stages: age, organ function, nutrition, and genetic variation. For example, elderly patients often require dosage adjustments because of decreased renal clearance. Technicians play a vital role in monitoring these parameters, ensuring that prescribed doses align with the patient's physiological capacity. Understanding pharmacokinetics allows technicians to anticipate drug interactions, manage timing between doses, and recognize when formulation changes are necessary. It transforms the act of dispensing into a scientifically informed contribution to therapeutic success.

Routes and Forms of Drug Administration

The route of administration determines both the onset and intensity of a drug's effect. Common routes include oral, parenteral, topical, inhalation, and transdermal delivery. Each route demands specific preparation and handling techniques to maintain sterility and effectiveness. Oral medications are convenient but subject to first-pass metabolism, which can reduce bioavailability. Parenteral routes, such as intravenous or intramuscular injection, bypass the digestive system and deliver rapid systemic action, but they require strict aseptic technique. Topical and transdermal preparations provide localized or sustained systemic absorption, while inhaled medications offer targeted delivery to the respiratory tract. Pharmacy technicians must understand the implications of each route when selecting dosage forms, calculating concentrations, and counseling patients. For example, sustained-release tablets should never be crushed, as doing so may alter absorption rates and cause toxicity. Recognizing the relationship between formulation and route ensures that every medication functions as intended, preserving both efficacy and patient safety.

Dosage Calculations and Accuracy in Therapy

Precision in dosage calculation represents the most critical technical skill in pharmacy practice. Whether converting between units, calculating concentration ratios, or determining infusion rates, accuracy prevents both underdosing and overdose. Dimensional analysis provides a universal method for solving dosage problems without reliance on memorized formulas, ensuring consistency across varying medication orders. Technicians must master conversions within and between the metric, apothecary, and household systems, applying these calculations to real prescriptions under supervision. Pediatric and geriatric populations require particular care, as small errors can have significant physiological consequences. Verification processes—double-checking calculations, using calibrated devices, and documenting results—transform arithmetic into professional diligence. The integration of technology, such as automated dispensing and dosage calculators, aids precision but never replaces human oversight. A certified technician's understanding of calculation principles upholds the central ethical promise of pharmacy: to deliver the correct medication in the correct dose to the correct patient at the correct time.

Adverse Drug Reactions and Side Effect Management

Adverse drug reactions (ADRs) encompass all unintended, harmful effects resulting from therapeutic use of medications. These may range from mild discomfort to severe systemic toxicity. Understanding ADRs allows technicians to recognize early warning signs and respond appropriately under pharmacist supervision. Factors contributing to adverse reactions include allergies, interactions, genetic predispositions, and improper dosing. Reporting systems, such as institutional incident logs and national pharmacovigilance programs, rely on the technician's vigilance in documenting suspected events. Management of ADRs often requires discontinuation, substitution, or dosage adjustment, coordinated between the pharmacist and prescriber. Patient education also plays a preventive role; technicians help reinforce adherence to dosing schedules and awareness of potential symptoms. By maintaining awareness of drug-specific risks—such as nephrotoxicity, hepatotoxicity, or hypersensitivity—technicians actively reduce harm. The responsibility extends beyond observation to participation in creating a safer medication environment through knowledge, communication, and ethical action.

Drug Interactions and Compatibility Considerations

Drug interactions occur when one substance alters the effect of another, either enhancing, diminishing, or transforming its therapeutic outcome. These interactions may be pharmacokinetic, affecting absorption or metabolism, or pharmacodynamic, influencing receptor response. For example, combining anticoagulants with certain antibiotics can increase bleeding risk, while antacids may reduce absorption of oral medications. Pharmacy technicians are essential in identifying such risks through careful review of patient profiles and medication histories. Compatibility also extends to compounded preparations—mixing incompatible drugs can cause precipitation or inactivation. Electronic databases and interaction-checking software support this process, but understanding the principles behind these warnings ensures informed judgment. Communication with pharmacists and other healthcare professionals transforms detection into prevention. Recognizing and managing interactions demonstrates the technician's active role in safeguarding therapeutic integrity, ensuring that every combination dispensed contributes positively to patient health rather than compromising it.

Patient Education and Adherence to Therapy

Successful drug therapy depends not only on prescribing and dispensing but also on the patient's adherence to instructions. Pharmacy technicians often serve as the bridge between clinical directives and patient understanding. They reinforce dosing schedules, clarify administration techniques, and emphasize the importance of completing prescribed courses, particularly with antibiotics or chronic disease medications. Barriers to adherence include complex regimens, side effects, cost, and misunderstanding of instructions. Technicians can mitigate these by providing clear explanations, using visual aids, and ensuring that labeling matches literacy levels. Encouraging open dialogue helps patients express concerns, enabling the pharmacy team to adjust therapy when needed. In patient-centered care, education transforms compliance into collaboration. When patients understand why and how medications work, adherence improves, outcomes strengthen, and the pharmacist-technician partnership fulfills its ultimate goal—empowering individuals to manage their health responsibly.

Drug Storage, Stability, and Disposal

Proper storage conditions preserve drug stability and therapeutic effectiveness. Temperature, humidity, light, and contamination can degrade active ingredients, leading to reduced potency or harmful by-products. Technicians are responsible for monitoring storage environments, maintaining refrigeration logs, and following manufacturer guidelines. Stability also determines beyond-use dates for compounded preparations, which must be labeled accurately to prevent expired use. Disposal regulations protect both public safety and the environment. Controlled substances require witnessed destruction under documented procedures, while hazardous medications follow strict waste management protocols. In community settings, technicians often educate patients on safe disposal of unused drugs to prevent misuse or accidental ingestion. Each step—from storage to final disposal—reflects a continuum of care rooted in both science and responsibility. By maintaining environmental control and regulatory compliance, technicians preserve not just medication quality but also the integrity of the healthcare system.

The Technician's Role in Therapeutic Optimization

Therapeutic optimization refers to achieving the best possible clinical outcome for each patient through the precise use of medications. Technicians support this process by managing workflow efficiency, ensuring medication availability, and monitoring for adherence or duplication. Their role includes verifying refill patterns that may indicate misuse or underuse and flagging potential therapy gaps for pharmacist review. In institutional settings, technicians assist in collecting patient histories and reconciling medications during transitions of care—critical steps in preventing therapeutic error. Collaboration with pharmacists transforms routine dispensing into active contribution to clinical decision-making. As healthcare moves toward personalized medicine, technicians must adapt to new data systems, pharmacogenomic insights, and evolving drug protocols. Their combination of technical skill and ethical awareness ensures that therapy remains both effective and individualized. The certified technician thus functions not only as a support professional but as an essential partner in achieving the highest standards of pharmaceutical care.

Drug Classifications and Therapeutic Categories

Understanding drug classifications and therapeutic categories is fundamental for pharmacy technicians, as medications are grouped according to their therapeutic use, mechanism of action, or chemical structure. Drugs may be classified into broad therapeutic categories such as antihypertensives, antibiotics, analgesics, antidiabetics, antidepressants, and anticoagulants. Within each category, medications share common therapeutic goals but may differ in potency, dosing, or adverse effect profiles. For example, antihypertensives include multiple subclasses such as beta blockers, ACE inhibitors, calcium channel blockers, and diuretics, each working through distinct mechanisms to lower blood pressure. Technicians must recognize common brand and generic names within these categories to reduce dispensing errors and improve workflow efficiency. Awareness of look-alike and sound-alike medications is especially important in preventing selection mistakes. Drug classification knowledge also assists technicians in identifying potential storage requirements, such as refrigeration for certain biologics or controlled storage for scheduled medications. While pharmacy technicians do not provide clinical recommendations, understanding therapeutic categories enhances communication with pharmacists and supports accurate prescription processing. Familiarity with drug groupings also aids in recognizing common indications and typical dosage forms. Strong foundational knowledge of classifications ensures improved safety, accuracy, and professional competence within pharmacy operations.

Pharmacokinetics and Pharmacodynamics

Pharmacokinetics and pharmacodynamics describe how drugs move through and affect the body. Pharmacokinetics involves absorption, distribution, metabolism, and excretion. Absorption refers to how a drug enters the bloodstream, which may vary based on route of administration such as oral, topical, intravenous, or inhalation. Distribution describes how the medication travels through tissues and organs. Metabolism primarily occurs in the liver, where enzymes convert drugs into active or inactive metabolites. Excretion typically occurs through the kidneys but may also involve bile, sweat, or respiration. Pharmacodynamics explains how the drug interacts with receptors to produce therapeutic effects. This includes mechanisms such as receptor binding, enzyme inhibition, or alteration of cellular function. Factors such as age, body weight, organ function, and genetic variation can influence both pharmacokinetics and pharmacodynamics. Technicians must understand these concepts to appreciate why dosing adjustments may be required in pediatric, geriatric, or renal-impaired patients. Awareness of onset, peak, and duration of action supports proper medication scheduling and patient counseling by the pharmacist. While technicians do not determine dosing regimens, understanding how medications behave in the body reinforces safe handling and accurate processing of prescriptions.

Routes of Administration and Dosage Forms

Medications are available in various routes of administration and dosage forms, each designed to achieve specific therapeutic effects and accommodate patient needs. Common routes include oral, topical, inhalation, subcutaneous, intramuscular, intravenous, ophthalmic, otic, rectal, and transdermal. Oral dosage forms include tablets, capsules, liquids, and suspensions, each requiring proper labeling and measurement accuracy. Extended-release and enteric-coated formulations must not be crushed or altered due to modified release mechanisms. Topical preparations include creams, ointments, and patches designed for localized or systemic absorption. Parenteral medications require sterile preparation and precise technique in institutional settings. Inhalers and nebulized solutions deliver medication directly to the respiratory tract for rapid effect. Pharmacy technicians must recognize dosage form abbreviations and ensure correct product selection during dispensing. Some medications are available in multiple strengths and forms, requiring careful verification to prevent errors. Storage conditions may vary depending on dosage form, with certain injectables requiring refrigeration. Understanding routes and forms enhances accuracy, prevents substitution mistakes, and ensures that patients receive medications as prescribed. Knowledge of dosage form characteristics supports safe and efficient pharmacy operations.

Adverse Drug Reactions and Drug Interactions

Adverse drug reactions and drug interactions are critical considerations in medication therapy. Adverse reactions may range from mild side effects, such as nausea or dizziness, to severe allergic responses or life-threatening anaphylaxis. Some reactions are predictable based on pharmacologic action, while others are idiosyncratic or immune-mediated. Pharmacy technicians must document reported allergies accurately and alert pharmacists to potential concerns. Drug interactions occur when one medication alters the effect of another, potentially increasing toxicity or reducing therapeutic benefit. Interactions may also occur between drugs and foods, supplements, or herbal products. For example, certain antibiotics may interact with oral contraceptives, and anticoagulants may be affected by dietary vitamin intake. Technicians assist in gathering complete medication histories and entering data accurately into pharmacy systems that generate interaction alerts for pharmacist review. Awareness of high-alert medications and common interaction risks enhances vigilance during prescription processing. While clinical evaluation is the pharmacist's responsibility, technician attentiveness to allergy documentation and accurate data entry plays a key role in preventing medication-related harm. Recognizing the importance of adverse reactions and interactions reinforces patient safety and supports collaborative pharmacy practice.

Chapter 4: Dispensing Process

Prescription and Medication Order Intake

The dispensing process begins with accurate and lawful receipt of a prescription or medication order. At this stage, the pharmacy technician must verify that all essential components are present: patient identification, prescriber credentials, drug name, dosage form, strength, quantity, and instructions for use. This step transforms a clinical decision into an actionable order and requires careful interpretation to prevent miscommunication or error. Intake also involves confirming insurance or billing details, ensuring regulatory compliance, and recognizing potential irregularities that warrant clarification. In hospital settings, medication orders may originate electronically, whereas community pharmacies may handle handwritten prescriptions that demand additional scrutiny. The technician's role is to ensure that every order entering the workflow is complete, legible, and authentic. Effective intake establishes the foundation for all subsequent tasks, aligning operational precision with legal and ethical responsibility. A vigilant approach at this point prevents costly errors downstream and demonstrates the technician's integral contribution to patient safety.

Data Entry and Verification Accuracy

Once the prescription has been accepted, data entry transforms handwritten or digital information into a verified record within the pharmacy management system. Precision at this stage is critical because typographical errors or misinterpretation of abbreviations can lead to incorrect medication selection or dosing. Standard operating procedures require technicians to cross-check entries against the original prescription, confirming drug name, strength, and directions. In many institutions, barcoding and automated data capture enhance accuracy, but human oversight remains indispensable. Verification involves secondary review by another technician or pharmacist to ensure integrity of data before dispensing proceeds. Errors identified early prevent downstream waste and protect patients from harm. Accurate entry also supports billing, insurance claims, and regulatory reporting. The technician's meticulousness demonstrates professionalism and safeguards the reliability of pharmacy records. Data integrity at this stage exemplifies the blend of technical skill and ethical diligence that defines excellence in pharmacy operations.

Product Selection and Preparation

Selecting the correct product requires both knowledge and attention to detail. The technician must confirm that the chosen medication matches the prescriber's intent in name, strength, dosage form, and manufacturer when substitution is authorized. Errors can occur between look-alike or sound-alike medications, making barcode verification and physical label checks essential. Preparation may involve counting, measuring, compounding, or reconstituting medications according to established procedures. Each task demands precision and adherence to sanitation standards. For sterile preparations, technicians must follow aseptic technique within controlled environments such as laminar airflow hoods. Every label affixed must accurately convey drug name, directions, and auxiliary warnings. The process transforms raw pharmaceutical stock into individualized therapy, merging mechanical accuracy with human judgment. The technician's disciplined approach ensures that every medication leaving the preparation area represents the highest standard of care—safe, correct, and fully aligned with professional and legal expectations.

Compounding and Aseptic Technique

Compounding involves the preparation of customized medications when commercially available products do not meet specific patient needs. This may include adjusting dosage forms, combining ingredients, or producing sterile formulations. Aseptic technique is the cornerstone of compounding safety, preventing microbial contamination that could harm patients. Technicians performing sterile compounding must undergo rigorous training and competency assessment. Procedures such as hand hygiene, use of personal protective equipment, and maintenance of laminar airflow workbenches are non-negotiable. Measurements must be precise, with all calculations verified independently. Documentation records every ingredient, lot number, and expiration date to ensure traceability. Errors in compounding can have serious consequences, making attention to detail an ethical as well as technical duty. Adherence to established standards, such as those defined by pharmacopeial guidelines, ensures product integrity. The compounding process illustrates how scientific accuracy, regulatory compliance, and moral responsibility converge in the daily work of pharmacy technicians.

Labeling, Packaging, and Auxiliary Information

The label on a dispensed medication serves as the primary communication link between the pharmacy and the patient. It must clearly state the patient's name, medication identity, dosage instructions, and any relevant warnings. Legibility and completeness are not merely procedural—they are legal requirements. Technicians ensure that each label corresponds exactly to the verified prescription, avoiding typographical or transpositional errors. Auxiliary labels provide supplementary guidance, such as storage conditions or potential side effects. Packaging also contributes to safety, protecting medication from contamination, moisture, and light. For controlled substances, tamper-evident packaging is required. The presentation of the final product influences adherence; a well-labeled, clearly organized package helps patients understand and trust their therapy. Through meticulous labeling and packaging, the technician fulfills both an educational and protective role, transforming a clinical order into a safe, user-friendly product ready for patient use.

Pharmacist Verification and Quality Check

Before any medication is released, it undergoes a final verification by the pharmacist. The technician's responsibility is to prepare a complete and accurate product for review. This step represents the quality checkpoint where clinical and technical oversight converge. The pharmacist assesses appropriateness, dosing accuracy, and potential interactions, while the technician confirms that the physical product, label, and documentation align with the order. Open communication during verification ensures that discrepancies are addressed promptly. This collaborative process underscores the shared accountability inherent in pharmacy practice: technicians maintain precision in preparation, and pharmacists apply clinical judgment in approval. Together, they embody a safety net that protects patients from harm. Verification also serves as a learning opportunity, reinforcing the technician's professional development through feedback and correction. The process exemplifies teamwork grounded in mutual respect and shared ethical commitment to patient well-being.

Dispensing and Patient Counseling Support

Dispensing transforms the verified medication into a tangible therapeutic outcome for the patient. The technician ensures that the correct product, quantity, and label reach the intended individual. At the point of handover, technicians assist pharmacists by confirming identity, reviewing packaging integrity, and providing educational materials. While direct counseling is performed by pharmacists, technicians reinforce understanding by clarifying instructions and answering procedural questions within their scope. Communication must remain empathetic and professional, maintaining patient confidentiality at all times. The dispensing counter represents both the end of one process and the beginning of another—the patient's journey toward adherence and healing. By ensuring accuracy, confidentiality, and clear communication, technicians uphold the profession's promise to deliver medications safely and responsibly. Every interaction reinforces public trust in the pharmacy as a place of competence, integrity, and care.

Inventory Control and Storage Management

Efficient inventory control underpins the entire dispensing process. Technicians are responsible for monitoring stock levels, checking expiration dates, and ensuring that medications are stored under appropriate conditions. Proper inventory management prevents shortages, reduces waste, and maintains product integrity. Systems for automated tracking and reorder alerts support this function but depend on accurate data entry and human verification. Controlled substances require additional record-keeping and restricted access, ensuring compliance with regulatory standards. Rotation of stock—first in, first out—minimizes loss through expiration. Temperature logs, calibration checks, and visual inspections confirm environmental stability. Through organized storage, technicians facilitate quick retrieval, reduce dispensing errors, and maintain an efficient workflow. Effective inventory management demonstrates foresight and professionalism, ensuring that every prescription can be filled promptly without compromising quality or legality.

Documentation, Record Retention, and Audit Readiness

Documentation provides the legal and professional evidence of every dispensing transaction. Accurate records ensure accountability and traceability, allowing audits to confirm compliance with law and policy. Technicians are responsible for recording lot numbers, quantities dispensed, and any incidents or corrective actions. Record retention timelines vary by jurisdiction but universally reflect the principle that transparency sustains trust. Electronic documentation has improved accessibility and reduced duplication, yet it introduces the responsibility of maintaining digital security. Regular audits verify accuracy and identify process gaps. Preparedness for such reviews demonstrates organizational maturity. Each record, whether handwritten or electronic, tells the story of a technician's diligence and the pharmacy's integrity. Proper documentation transforms routine dispensing into a documented assurance of safety and compliance—a tangible reflection of the profession's ethical and legal foundations.

Continuous Improvement in Dispensing Practice

Dispensing excellence is achieved not through static adherence to rules but through continuous reflection and improvement. Technicians must remain receptive to innovation, whether through automation, barcode scanning, or evolving software platforms. Error reports and patient feedback provide valuable data for system enhancement. Participating in quality-improvement meetings, technicians contribute firsthand insights into workflow efficiency and risk reduction. Education remains a cornerstone; ongoing training ensures that skills evolve alongside industry standards. Improvement also involves humility—the willingness to analyze mistakes and convert them into lessons for collective advancement. The culture of continuous improvement transforms dispensing from a repetitive task into a dynamic process of professional growth. By committing to learning, reflection, and innovation, pharmacy technicians help sustain a system that is both safe and adaptable to future healthcare challenges.

Chapter 5: Medication and Patient Safety and Quality Assurance

Foundations of Medication Safety

Medication safety represents the core mission of pharmacy practice—the prevention of errors that could harm patients or undermine therapeutic outcomes. The concept extends beyond avoiding mistakes to building a culture that prioritizes vigilance, accountability, and continuous learning. Pharmacy technicians play a pivotal role in operationalizing safety through adherence to standardized workflows, double-check systems, and communication protocols. Every stage of the medication-use process, from procurement to administration, contains potential hazards that must be anticipated and managed. Safety begins with knowledge: understanding drug names, packaging similarities, and potential interactions enables technicians to recognize risk before it manifests. It also requires ethical integrity—a willingness to question inconsistencies and seek clarification rather than assume correctness. The foundation of safety is trust: trust between patients, pharmacists, and technicians that every medication prepared has been handled with care and verified for accuracy. This trust is earned daily through precision, professionalism, and unwavering attention to detail.

The Culture of Safety in Pharmacy Practice

A strong safety culture transforms isolated safeguards into an enduring organizational mindset. In such an environment, all staff members—pharmacists, technicians, and support personnel—share a collective responsibility for preventing harm. Communication is open, errors are reported without fear of punishment, and learning replaces blame. The Institute for Safe Medication Practices advocates a systems-based approach, emphasizing that most errors arise from flawed processes rather than individual negligence. Technicians reinforce this culture by adhering to protocols, participating in safety meetings, and modeling consistency in their actions. Leadership within the pharmacy fosters safety by promoting transparency, recognizing diligence, and investing in continuous education. Over time, this culture permeates every aspect of the pharmacy's operation, influencing how medications are labeled, stored, and verified. A strong safety culture does not eliminate risk but transforms how it is managed—proactively, collaboratively, and compassionately. Through this shared commitment, the pharmacy evolves into a place where every decision reflects the collective duty to protect patients.

Identifying and Reporting Medication Errors

Medication errors can occur at any stage—prescribing, transcribing, dispensing, or administration. Detecting and reporting them promptly prevents recurrence and saves lives. Pharmacy technicians are often the first to notice discrepancies, whether through mismatched dosages, unclear labels, or incomplete records. Effective reporting systems rely on honesty and detail; technicians must document what occurred, when, and under what circumstances. Reports should focus on system improvement, not personal blame. Many organizations maintain confidential or anonymous reporting mechanisms that encourage participation. Documentation of near misses is equally valuable because it exposes weaknesses before harm occurs. Follow-up analysis identifies root causes, leading to revised procedures or additional training. The act of reporting is both professional and ethical, demonstrating commitment to continuous improvement. By transforming error recognition into a learning opportunity, pharmacy technicians turn challenges into catalysts for safer practice and stronger teamwork across all levels of healthcare delivery.

Root Cause Analysis and Preventive Strategies

Root cause analysis (RCA) is a systematic method used to investigate why an error occurred and how to prevent recurrence. It shifts attention from individual fault to process vulnerability. When a medication error or near miss is reported, an RCA team examines contributing factors such as workflow design, staffing levels, communication barriers, and environmental conditions. Pharmacy technicians often provide essential insight because they understand daily operational realities. Their perspective helps identify practical solutions, such as reorganizing workspaces or standardizing labeling formats. Preventive strategies may include double verification for high-alert drugs, color-coded storage, or enhanced staff training. The ultimate goal of RCA is not to assign blame but to strengthen the system. Implemented effectively, these strategies create a feedback loop that fosters continuous learning and resilience. Through participation in RCA, technicians become active architects of safer systems, transforming experience into prevention and contributing meaningfully to the evolution of patient-centered care.

High-Alert Medications and Risk Mitigation

Certain medications carry a heightened risk of causing severe harm if used incorrectly. These high-alert drugs—such as anticoagulants, opioids, insulin, and chemotherapy agents—require special handling and monitoring. Pharmacy technicians play a critical role in identifying, labeling, and managing these substances according to strict institutional guidelines. Risk mitigation includes segregated storage, independent double checks, and clear documentation of preparation and dispensing steps. Each action reduces the likelihood of accidental interchange or dosing error. Understanding the pharmacology and potential consequences of high-alert medications reinforces the technician's awareness of their responsibility. Education and simulation exercises strengthen preparedness for unusual scenarios, such as emergency dosing or contamination control. The safe handling of these drugs exemplifies the harmony between precision and ethical duty. Technicians who master risk mitigation techniques embody the profession's central promise—to preserve life through meticulous care and unwavering attention to safety protocols.

Infection Control and Sterile Practices

Preventing contamination is an inseparable element of medication safety. Infection control procedures protect both patients and healthcare workers from transmissible pathogens during medication preparation and handling. Pharmacy technicians, especially those involved in compounding or sterile product preparation, must maintain aseptic technique as a daily discipline. Proper hand hygiene, gowning, and equipment disinfection minimize the risk of microbial introduction. Controlled environments, such as cleanrooms or laminar airflow hoods, require routine monitoring for particulate counts and airflow integrity. The CDC and professional compounding standards outline clear procedures for maintaining sterility, emphasizing that environmental vigilance equals clinical protection. Failure to follow these practices can lead to outbreaks, product recalls, and patient harm. Therefore, infection control is not ancillary to pharmacy—it is central to its ethical and professional purpose. By treating every dose as a potential safeguard or threat, technicians reinforce the sacred trust that defines safe pharmaceutical care.

Patient Safety and Communication Practices

Communication remains one of the most powerful tools in ensuring patient safety. Miscommunication between prescribers, pharmacists, and technicians often leads to preventable errors. Clear verbal and written exchanges, standardized abbreviations, and active listening mitigate this risk. Technicians must confirm patient identity using multiple identifiers before dispensing medications, and they should never assume clarity in an ambiguous order. Patients themselves are critical partners in safety; educating them about medication purpose, appearance, and proper use reduces confusion. Cultural sensitivity and language assistance further enhance understanding. Within the pharmacy, communication extends to documentation—accurate, timely notes that inform others of changes or concerns. Every message transmitted accurately contributes to the reliability of the healthcare system. In this sense, communication is both a clinical skill and a moral responsibility. When technicians communicate with precision and empathy, they embody the essence of patient-centered safety.

Continuous Quality Improvement Programs

Quality assurance is the structured, ongoing evaluation of pharmacy processes to ensure optimal outcomes. Continuous Quality Improvement (CQI) programs provide the framework for detecting, analyzing, and correcting system weaknesses. These programs rely on measurable indicators such as error rates, turnaround times, and patient satisfaction. Pharmacy technicians contribute by collecting data, participating in audits, and implementing revised workflows. CQI fosters collaboration, uniting clinical and operational staff around the shared goal of safer, more efficient service. Feedback from these programs often leads to procedural refinements—new labeling standards, enhanced storage design, or improved documentation methods. The strength of CQI lies in its iterative nature: assessment, improvement, and reassessment form an unbroken cycle. For technicians, participation in CQI builds professional insight and fosters a proactive mindset. By engaging in these efforts, they affirm that quality is not a static achievement but an evolving commitment to excellence.

Risk Management and Regulatory Compliance

Risk management encompasses the identification, evaluation, and control of potential threats to patient safety, legal compliance, and institutional integrity. In pharmacy, this involves strict adherence to policies for medication storage, handling, and record keeping. Technicians act as the first line of defense by recognizing hazards—expired stock, incomplete documentation, or unsafe workflow patterns—and reporting them for correction. Regulatory compliance reinforces risk management by aligning operations with national and local standards. Audits and inspections serve not as punitive measures but as opportunities for validation and improvement. Failure to comply can result in legal penalties or loss of certification, but proactive compliance strengthens professional credibility. Effective risk management transforms rules into daily habits, ensuring that each action within the pharmacy contributes to a stable and trustworthy system. Through diligence and ethical awareness, technicians protect not only their patients but the integrity of their profession.

Ethical Dimensions of Patient Safety

Ethics and safety are inseparable in pharmacy practice. Every decision made by a technician reflects a moral judgment about the value of human life and the responsibility to protect it. Ethical safety involves more than rule-following—it requires empathy, honesty, and moral courage. Technicians must be willing to speak up when they identify unsafe conditions or questionable instructions, even when doing so challenges hierarchy. Confidentiality, respect, and informed consent form the moral framework for all interactions. The ethical dimension extends beyond compliance into compassion: understanding that behind every vial or tablet lies a person placing trust in the system. The integrity of that trust depends on moral consistency as much as on technical accuracy. When technicians approach safety with ethical conviction, they transform procedural competence into moral excellence. Patient safety thus becomes not merely a professional requirement but a reflection of humanity's collective respect for life.

Advancing Safety Through Education and Innovation

The pursuit of medication safety evolves continuously through education, technology, and innovation. Automation, electronic prescribing, and barcode verification have reduced human error, but their effectiveness depends on informed operators. Ongoing professional education ensures that technicians remain competent in new systems and aware of emerging risks. Simulation training and case-based learning cultivate judgment under realistic conditions. Innovation also includes process redesign—streamlining communication channels, integrating decision-support software, and optimizing workspace ergonomics. Technicians who embrace lifelong learning become catalysts for progress, bridging traditional practice with modern advancement. Education sustains vigilance, while innovation expands capability. Together they embody the forward motion of the profession: a continuous ascent toward safer, smarter, and more compassionate care. Through dedication to both knowledge and adaptability, pharmacy technicians secure their role as guardians of patient safety in an ever-changing healthcare landscape.

Chapter 6 – Practice Questions

Questions (1-100)

Q1. Which of the following tasks is within the scope of practice for a pharmacy technician?

A. Counseling patients about side effects
B. Selecting appropriate drug therapy
C. Preparing and labeling medications
D. Modifying a patient's prescription dosage

Q2. In a pharmacy setting, which responsibility best demonstrates professional communication by a technician?

A. Ignoring a patient's complaint to avoid confrontation
B. Discussing prescription details in a public area
C. Maintaining confidentiality during interactions
D. Providing dosage instructions to patients

Q3. What is the primary reason pharmacy technicians must verify patient identifiers before dispensing medication?

A. To improve workflow speed
B. To ensure medication safety and accuracy
C. To comply with insurance regulations
D. To minimize paperwork

Q4. When receiving a new prescription, which of the following should a technician immediately verify before processing?

A. The patient's insurance deductible
B. The prescribing physician's license number
C. The completeness and legibility of the order
D. The patient's medical diagnosis

Q5. Which scenario shows a technician acting outside their legal scope of practice?

A. Recommending an OTC product for a patient's rash
B. Entering refill information into the computer system
C. Compounding a cream as directed by a pharmacist
D. Counting and labeling tablets

Q6. A pharmacy technician must maintain accurate inventory records primarily to:

A. Track profits and losses
B. Prevent medication shortages and errors
C. Assist in advertising promotions
D. Support the marketing department

Q7. Which task is part of the pharmacy workflow handled by technicians?

A. Counseling a patient about drug interactions
B. Verifying prescription accuracy
C. Counting, pouring, or packaging medications
D. Selecting drug therapy for chronic conditions

Q8. Which of the following describes an essential ethical duty of pharmacy technicians?

A. Prioritizing workload convenience
B. Protecting patient confidentiality
C. Discussing medical conditions with other customers
D. Adjusting prescriptions for faster service

Q9. The technician should notify the pharmacist immediately if:

A. The patient requests information about side effects

B. A refill is due next week
C. A patient asks for a receipt
D. The patient requests a change in dosage

Q10. Why must pharmacy technicians maintain a clean and organized workspace?
A. To create a comfortable environment
B. To prevent medication contamination or mix-ups
C. To make the area visually appealing
D. To speed up insurance processing

Q11. During prescription entry, a technician notices an illegible doctor's handwriting. The technician should:
A. Guess based on the patient's medication history
B. Clarify with the pharmacist before processing
C. Contact the prescriber directly without permission
D. Leave the field blank and continue

Q12. Which of the following demonstrates proper teamwork in a pharmacy?
A. Ignoring tasks that belong to others
B. Sharing updates about prescription issues
C. Refusing to communicate with staff
D. Working independently on all tasks

Q13. Why must technicians confirm medication expiration dates?
A. To ensure drugs meet safety and potency standards
B. To reduce inventory costs
C. To track supplier performance
D. To satisfy patient curiosity

Q14. Which duty requires extra attention to detail from technicians?
A. Cleaning shelves
B. Entering prescription data
C. Scheduling staff shifts
D. Designing advertisements

Q15. Why must pharmacy technicians wear identification badges?
A. To advertise pharmacy services
B. To display personal achievements
C. To maintain professional transparency and accountability
D. To comply with sales requirements

Q16. What should a pharmacy technician do if a patient presents a prescription for a controlled substance?
A. Verify the patient's identification
B. Ignore the prescription and inform the pharmacist
C. Ask the patient for the physician's contact details
D. Suggest alternative medications

Q17. A patient requests to pick up a prescription but cannot provide identification. What should the technician do?
A. Ask the pharmacist to verify the identity
B. Inform the patient they cannot receive the medication
C. Offer the medication without asking for ID
D. Contact the prescribing doctor for verification

Q18. A pharmacy technician is asked to prepare a prescription that includes an allergy warning. The technician should:

A. Ignore the warning and proceed with preparation
B. Ask the patient for their allergy history
C. Inform the pharmacist about the allergy note
D. Contact the physician for clarification

Q19. When handling prescriptions for pediatric patients, the technician must:
A. Verify the dosage based on the patient's weight
B. Suggest a smaller dose to the pharmacist
C. Refill the prescription without confirming with the pharmacist
D. Ignore age-based dosage adjustments

Q20. When restocking medications on the shelf, a pharmacy technician should:
A. Place expired medications in the front
B. Leave expired medications on the shelf until they are requested
C. Rotate stock to ensure the newest medications are in front
D. Ignore the shelf labeling system

Q21. What is the technician's role in drug recalls?
A. Destroy recalled medications
B. Inform the patient of the recall directly
C. Contact the manufacturer for further instructions
D. Remove recalled drugs from the shelf and notify the pharmacist

Q22. If a patient refuses a medication due to a perceived side effect, the technician should:
A. Tell the patient they are wrong about the side effect
B. Offer them a different drug without consulting the pharmacist
C. Inform the pharmacist about the patient's concern
D. Ignore the refusal and continue dispensing

Q23. How should a technician handle a prescription for a patient who is allergic to a specific medication ingredient?
A. Dispense the medication after informing the pharmacist
B. Call the patient's doctor for approval to change the ingredient
C. Tell the patient to try the medication anyway
D. Ignore the allergy note and proceed with dispensing

Q24. A technician notices a prescription has an unusual dosage form, such as a liquid instead of tablets. The technician should:
A. Process the prescription as usual
B. Verify the dosage form with the pharmacist before dispensing
C. Tell the patient the prescription is incorrect
D. Refuse to process the prescription

Q25. When providing medication counseling to a patient, what must a pharmacy technician ensure?
A. That they prescribe the medication for the patient
B. That they explain potential side effects in detail
C. That they follow the instructions of the pharmacist
D. That they offer medical advice on treatment options

Q26. Which of the following is the primary responsibility of a pharmacy technician when processing a prescription?
A. Selecting the drug dosage
B. Performing clinical assessments
C. Preparing medications for pharmacist review
D. Prescribing medication changes

Q27. Which action demonstrates a pharmacy technician's adherence to patient safety protocols?

A. Recommending an OTC product for a patient's symptoms
B. Double-checking medication labels before dispensing
C. Ignoring labeling instructions if they're unclear
D. Working without consulting the pharmacist

Q28. How should a pharmacy technician handle a medication error that has already been dispensed to a patient?

A. Ignore the error and hope the patient does not notice
B. Immediately inform the pharmacist and document the error
C. Ask the patient to return the medication on their own
D. Change the medication without telling the pharmacist

Q29. A pharmacy technician should always verify a patient's allergy information before dispensing medications because:

A. It helps avoid medications with potentially harmful allergens
B. It ensures the patient gets the cheapest drug
C. It speeds up the dispensing process
D. It is not required unless the patient asks

Q30. When a technician notices a prescription for a controlled substance, what is their first action?

A. Process the prescription as usual
B. Verify the patient's identity and ensure compliance with regulations
C. Consult the physician for dosage changes
D. Ask the patient to leave the pharmacy

Q31. Why is it important for pharmacy technicians to stay current with drug formulations and dosages?

A. To recommend the best drugs for patients
B. To ensure correct medications are dispensed in the proper form
C. To suggest alternative drugs to patients
D. To minimize drug costs

Q32. What should a pharmacy technician do if a patient asks for a medication that is not on the pharmacy's formulary?

A. Dispense an alternative without consulting the pharmacist
B. Suggest a different medication and discuss with the pharmacist
C. Refuse to process the prescription
D. Immediately refer the patient to another pharmacy

Q33. Which of the following is the primary duty of a pharmacy technician when assisting the pharmacist with sterile compounding?

A. Conducting drug calculations
B. Selecting appropriate ingredients
C. Compounding medications and maintaining aseptic technique
D. Counseling patients on drug administration

Q34. How can pharmacy technicians contribute to preventing medication errors in a busy pharmacy environment?

A. By ignoring procedural protocols to save time
B. By working independently without consulting the pharmacist
C. By focusing on administrative tasks and leaving dispensing to pharmacists
D. By following prescribed procedures and double-checking medication orders

Q35. A pharmacy technician is preparing a prescription when they notice a discrepancy in the dosage prescribed. What should they do?

A. Adjust the dosage according to what seems appropriate
B. Proceed without addressing the discrepancy

C. Consult the pharmacist immediately for clarification
D. Inform the patient that the dosage is wrong

Q36. What is the purpose of patient counseling in the pharmacy setting?
A. To sell additional pharmacy services
B. To provide information about side effects and medication usage
C. To prescribe alternative medications
D. To collect feedback about pharmacy staff

Q37. Why should a pharmacy technician be aware of look-alike, sound-alike drugs?
A. To improve pharmacy sales
B. To avoid dispensing the wrong medication due to confusion
C. To choose the cheapest drug for patients
D. To recommend drugs with fewer side effects

Q38. Which of the following actions would NOT be considered a violation of HIPAA for a pharmacy technician?
A. Discussing a patient's medication in public
B. Reviewing a patient's prescription in private with the pharmacist
C. Writing down a patient's personal information in a public log
D. Sharing patient information with unauthorized individuals

Q39. When should a pharmacy technician request clarification from a pharmacist regarding a prescription?
A. When they are unsure of the medication's name
B. When the prescription is for an over-the-counter drug
C. When the patient requests a specific medication
D. When the technician is too busy to process the prescription

Q40. A pharmacy technician receives a prescription for a controlled substance. What should be verified before dispensing?
A. The patient's medical history
B. The dosage and formulation of the medication
C. The patient's ID and prescription validity
D. The pharmacy's stock levels

Q41. A pharmacy technician is asked to assist with sterile compounding. What is their role?
A. Prescribing medications for compounding
B. Counseling the patient on compounded medications
C. Managing patient appointments for compounding services
D. Preparing sterile compounds while adhering to aseptic techniques

Q42. Which of the following would be considered a violation of a pharmacy technician's professional ethics?
A. Correctly labeling medications
B. Following a pharmacist's instructions
C. Dispensing medication without a prescription
D. Documenting all medications accurately

Q43. Why is it important for pharmacy technicians to stay updated on new drug developments?
A. To recommend the latest drugs to patients
B. To ensure correct drug handling and dispensing
C. To improve personal job performance
D. To influence the pharmacy's purchasing decisions

Q44. What should a pharmacy technician do if they are uncertain about the correct drug for a prescription?

A. Guess based on previous knowledge
B. Consult the pharmacist for guidance
C. Proceed with dispensing without question
D. Ask a colleague for their opinion

Q45. When receiving a prescription from a doctor for a controlled substance, the pharmacy technician should:
A. Dispense the medication immediately
B. Verify the medication's cost for the patient
C. Ask the patient if they have used the drug before
D. Verify the patient's identity and ensure the prescription is complete

Q46. Why must a pharmacy technician verify the National Drug Code (NDC) before dispensing?
A. To ensure the correct manufacturer, strength, and dosage form are selected
B. To increase inventory turnover
C. To simplify shelf organization
D. To speed up cashier transactions

Q47. A prescription requires 250 mg of a medication, and the available tablets are 125 mg each. How many tablets should be dispensed per dose?
A. 1 tablet
B. 2 tablets
C. 3 tablets
D. 0.5 tablet

Q48. Why must a pharmacy technician compare the stock bottle label to the prescription label during filling?
A. To reduce printing errors
B. To confirm the correct drug and strength are selected
C. To verify insurance information
D. To organize shelves more efficiently

Q49. If a prescription calls for 5 mL of a 100 mg/5 mL suspension, how many milligrams will the patient receive per dose?
A. 5 mg
B. 20 mg
C. 100 mg
D. 500 mg

Q50. Why should a pharmacy technician check the expiration date before dispensing a medication?
A. To avoid inventory waste
B. To ensure the medication maintains safety and effectiveness
C. To rotate stock faster
D. To comply with store policy only

Q51. When processing a prescription for a controlled substance, which document must the pharmacy technician check?
A. Patient's insurance card
B. A valid photo ID
C. Patient's medical history
D. Prescription drug monitoring program (PDMP) report

Q52. Which of the following is an important responsibility for a pharmacy technician in inventory management?
A. Providing drug recommendations to patients
B. Stocking and rotating medications based on expiration dates

C. Counseling patients on drug usage
D. Writing prescription orders

Q53. When labeling a prescription, which of the following must be included?
A. The pharmacist's full name
B. The patient's date of birth
C. The drug's expiration date
D. The patient's payment method

Q54. Which of the following is an example of misbranding in a pharmacy?
A. Dispensing a medication without a prescription
B. Labeling a medication with incorrect dosage instructions
C. Administering a medication to the wrong patient
D. Verifying a prescription with the pharmacist

Q55. What should a pharmacy technician do if a patient is unable to understand the medication instructions on their label?
A. Refer the patient to a pharmacist for counselling
B. Provide the patient with a larger print label
C. Ask the patient to find another pharmacy
D. Provide the patient with a drug pamphlet

Q56. A pharmacy technician is required to maintain confidentiality in all of the following situations except:
A. Discussing patient information in private with the pharmacist
B. Talking to a colleague about a patient's medical history
C. Verifying patient details with authorized individuals
D. Informing the patient about their medication instructions

Q57. Why is it important for a pharmacy technician to understand drug interactions?
A. To recommend the best drugs to patients
B. To accurately label and dispense medications
C. To provide alternative medications to patients
D. To assist the pharmacist in preventing harmful interactions

Q58. How should a pharmacy technician handle a prescription for a medication with a black box warning?
A. Ignore the warning unless the patient asks about it
B. Discuss the warning with the pharmacist and ensure the patient is informed
C. Proceed with dispensing without consulting the pharmacist
D. Offer the patient a different drug

Q59. What is the best course of action if a patient requests a medication that is not in stock?
A. Dispense an alternative medication without consulting the pharmacist
B. Tell the patient to try another pharmacy
C. Notify the pharmacist and check for any alternatives or availability
D. Inform the patient that their medication will not be available

Q60. What action should a pharmacy technician take when they receive an expired medication from a supplier?
A. Dispense it anyway if there's no alternative
B. Return it to the supplier for a replacement
C. Keep it in stock until the expiration date passes
D. Sell it with a discount to customers

Q61. Why is it important for a pharmacy technician to know how to use drug reference materials?
A. To dispense medications without a prescription

B. To quickly answer patient questions about drug side effects
C. To accurately prepare and label medications with the correct information
D. To recommend specific drugs to patients

Q62. When should a pharmacy technician notify the pharmacist about a medication error?
A. When the technician notices the error while labeling the medication
B. Only if the patient complains about the medication
C. If the error occurs during the pharmacist's verification process
D. If the technician is unsure of the medication being dispensed

Q63. How should a pharmacy technician manage inventory for medications that require refrigeration?
A. Store them with room-temperature medications
B. Keep them in a designated refrigerator with appropriate temperature control
C. Keep them in the freezer for better preservation
D. Discard them if they've been refrigerated for more than 24 hours

Q64. What is the role of the pharmacy technician in handling hazardous drugs?
A. Dispensing the medication without protection
B. Ensuring that proper handling, storage, and disposal procedures are followed
C. Preparing hazardous drugs without any training
D. Giving the medication to patients without any protective equipment

Q65. If a pharmacy technician is asked to prepare a medication that requires reconstitution, what must they do?
A. Reconstitute the medication using any available solvent
B. Skip the reconstitution process
C. Guess the solvent needed based on similar medications
D. Follow the manufacturer's instructions for the proper solvent and method

Q66. What should a pharmacy technician do if a medication is found to be damaged during the dispensing process?
A. Dispense it anyway if the patient is in a hurry
B. Dispose of it immediately without informing anyone
C. Notify the pharmacist and place it in the designated area for damaged goods
D. Place it back on the shelf after examining it

Q67. When a prescription is written with no refills, what should the pharmacy technician do?
A. Dispense the medication and add refills for convenience
B. Ask the patient if they would like refills added
C. Process the prescription as written, without refills
D. Ignore the no-refill instruction

Q68. Which of the following is NOT an appropriate action for a pharmacy technician when handling patient records?
A. Reviewing patient records for medication history
B. Sharing patient details with unauthorized individuals
C. Ensuring patient records are stored securely
D. Ensuring records are updated with the most recent prescriptions

Q69. What should a pharmacy technician do if they notice a medication recall notice for a product they are about to dispense?
A. Continue dispensing the medication unless the patient complains
B. Immediately inform the pharmacist and remove the medication from stock
C. Offer the patient a substitute without consulting the pharmacist
D. Tell the patient to return to the pharmacy later

Q70. Which of the following is a key responsibility of a pharmacy technician when preparing a medication for a patient?
A. Adjusting the dosage based on the patient's request
B. Counseling the patient on medication interactions
C. Verifying the medication's correct dosage form and label
D. Prescribing medication refills
Q71. What should a pharmacy technician do if they find a medication error during the dispensing process?
A. Correct the error and dispense the medication
B. Report the error to the pharmacist and do not proceed with dispensing
C. Ignore the error if the patient is in a hurry
D. Notify the patient about the error without informing the pharmacist
Q72. When preparing a medication for a pediatric patient, why is it important to verify the child's weight before dispensing?
A. To ensure the child receives the correct medication dosage
B. To determine if the medication is age-appropriate
C. To verify that the medication is safe to use in children
D. To help reduce the overall cost of the medication
Q73. A patient presents a prescription for a narcotic, and the pharmacy technician notices an issue with the prescription. What should they do?
A. Dispense the medication and inform the pharmacist later
B. Process the prescription without questioning it
C. Alert the pharmacist and confirm the prescription's validity
D. Refuse to process the prescription altogether
Q74. What is the correct procedure for a pharmacy technician when handling medications with controlled access?
A. Dispense them without restrictions, as long as they are prescribed
B. Store them in any available space in the pharmacy
C. Keep them locked up and access them only when necessary
D. Allow patients to pick them up without any verification
Q75. What should a pharmacy technician do if they are unsure about a specific drug interaction for a prescription?
A. Guess based on the patient's medical history
B. Consult a drug reference or ask the pharmacist for guidance
C. Ignore the potential interaction if the patient seems fine
D. Proceed with dispensing the medication without consulting anyone
Q76. When a pharmacy technician is dispensing a medication that requires specialpecial storage, such as refrigeration, what must they ensure?
A. The medication is labeled for refrigeration but left at room temperature
B. The medication is stored in a controlled, appropriate environment
C. The medication is dispensed without concern for storage
D. The medication is stored next to other non-refrigerated medications
Q77. A patient presents a prescription for a high-risk medication. What should the pharmacy technician do to ensure the medication is dispensed safely?
A. Dispense the medication without verification
B. Ask the patient about previous doses taken
C. Verify the prescription with the pharmacist and double-check the dosage
D. Skip the verification process for time efficiency

Q78. When a medication is dispensed in a blister pack instead of a traditional bottle, the technician should:
A. Ignore the blister pack and use a bottle instead
B. Check the medication against the prescription and ensure the correct dose is in each blister
C. Return the blister pack to the manufacturer for repackaging
D. Add additional pills to the blister pack to ensure a full supply
Q79. What is the pharmacy technician's role in medication therapy management (MTM)?
A. To independently adjust a patient's medication regimen
B. To conduct detailed clinical assessments of the patient's health
C. To prescribe medications to patients with chronic conditions
D. To collect and review a patient's medication history for the pharmacist's review
Q80. A pharmacy technician receives a prescription for a patient with a known allergy to penicillin. What should the technician do?
A. Dispense the medication as directed without making any changes
B. Alert the pharmacist immediately to verify the medication and alternative treatments
C. Provide the patient with a medication that does not contain penicillin, without consulting the pharmacist
D. Ignore the allergy warning if the patient does not mention it again
Q81. When a pharmacy technician is handling hazardous medications, which of the following is required?
A. Wearing gloves only
B. Wearing protective equipment such as gowns and gloves
C. Wearing regular work clothes and avoiding direct contact
D. No special precautions are needed
Q82. What should a pharmacy technician do if they notice a medication shortage in the pharmacy?
A. Dispense an alternative medication without consulting the pharmacist
B. Inform the pharmacist about the shortage and check for available alternatives
C. Ignore the shortage and continue with the normal dispensing process
D. Tell the patient to wait until the medication is back in stock
Q83. A patient's prescription is missing the doctor's signature. What should the pharmacy technician do?
A. Proceed with dispensing the medication
B. Call the patient to sign the prescription
C. Inform the pharmacist about the missing signature and refrain from dispensing
D. Fill the prescription based on verbal instructions from the patient
Q84. In a pharmacy, why is it important for a technician to follow proper hand hygiene when handling medications?
A. To prevent medication contamination and ensure safety
B. To reduce workload and increase efficiency
C. To reduce costs of medications
D. To improve communication with patients
Q85. What is the correct procedure for handling a prescription for a controlled substance that is presented after normal business hours?
A. Dispense the medication immediately without verifying with a pharmacist
B. Wait until the next business day to process the prescription
C. Call the prescribing doctor for clarification and then dispense
D. Verify with the pharmacist and follow the applicable state or federal regulations

Q86. When should a pharmacy technician consult the pharmacist about a potential drug-drug interaction?
A. Only if the patient asks about side effects
B. When the technician notices a discrepancy in the prescription
C. If the technician is unsure about the potential effects of two medications
D. If the pharmacist requests the technician's help
Q87. Which of the following actions should a pharmacy technician take to maintain security of medications in the pharmacy?
A. Leave controlled substances out in the open for easy access
B. Lock up medications in designated secure areas when not in use
C. Allow patients to handle medications when browsing
D. Allow non-pharmacy personnel to access medication storage areas
Q88. If a pharmacy technician makes a mistake during the medication preparation process, what should they do?
A. Ignore the mistake and continue with the preparation
B. Inform the pharmacist and correct the mistake immediately
C. Ask the patient to return the medication
D. Proceed with the dispensing process and make a note of the error
Q89. When a medication is dispensed with special handling instructions, who is responsible for ensuring the instructions are communicated to the patient?
A. The pharmacy technician
B. The prescribing physician
C. The patient's family member
D. The pharmacist
Q90. A pharmacy technician is asked to process a prescription for a patient with multiple medications. What should they check?
A. Only the drug names
B. The medication interactions and dosage adjustments
C. The patient's medical history
D. The payment method
Q91. Which federal agency regulates the manufacture and distribution of controlled substances?
A. Food and Drug Administration (FDA)
B. Centers for Disease Control and Prevention (CDC)
C. Drug Enforcement Administration (DEA)
D. Federal Trade Commission (FTC)
Q92. The Controlled Substances Act (CSA) categorizes drugs based on which of the following criteria?
A. Manufacturer and dosage form
B. Medical use and potential for abuse
C. Cost and insurance coverage
D. Brand and generic status
Q93. Which DEA form is required to order Schedule II controlled substances?
A. DEA Form 222
B. DEA Form 41
C. DEA Form 106
D. DEA Form 224
Q94. A pharmacy technician notices a missing quantity of a Schedule II drug. What should be done first?
A. Destroy remaining stock immediately
B. File a DEA Form 41

C. Notify the pharmacist and file DEA Form 106
D. Contact the FDA directly
Q95. Schedule II controlled substances can be refilled how many times under federal law?
A. Once
B. Twice
C. Three times
D. Zero times
Q96. Which of the following best describes a Schedule III controlled substance?
A. High potential for abuse; no accepted medical use
B. Moderate potential for abuse; accepted medical use
C. Low potential for abuse; no accepted medical use
D. No abuse potential; unrestricted use
Q97. How long must pharmacies maintain DEA 222 forms and controlled substance records?
A. 1 year
B. 2 years
C. 3 years
D. 5 years
Q98. What is the maximum number of refills allowed for Schedule III or IV controlled substances?
A. 2 refills within 3 months
B. 10 refills within 12 months
C. Unlimited refills within 1 year
D. 5 refills within 6 months
Q99. Which act requires child-resistant packaging for prescription drugs?
A. Controlled Substances Act
B. Poison Prevention Packaging Act
C. Omnibus Budget Reconciliation Act
D. Food, Drug, and Cosmetic Act
Q100. Which of the following drugs is classified as a Schedule II substance?
A. Alprazolam
B. Diazepam
C. Hydrocodone
D. Pregabalin

Answer keys and Explanations (1-100)

Q1. Answer: C
Explanation: Preparing and labeling medications is a core technical responsibility of pharmacy technicians. This task involves accurately counting, measuring, and labeling medications as per the prescription, under the supervision of a pharmacist. This supports workflow, safety, and regulatory compliance. It is a technical function that does not require clinical decision-making, which is outside the technician's role.

Q2. Answer: C
Explanation: Maintaining confidentiality is a key aspect of professional communication in pharmacy practice. Pharmacy technicians must safeguard patient privacy and discuss medication-related information only in private, secure settings. This ensures patient trust, respects legal and ethical obligations (e.g., HIPAA), and contributes to the pharmacy's overall professionalism. Confidentiality is paramount in all healthcare interactions and strengthens the patient-care relationship.

Q3. Answer: B
Explanation: Verifying patient identifiers is crucial to ensuring the correct medication is dispensed to the correct patient. This process helps prevent potentially harmful medication errors, such as giving the wrong drug or dosage. Patient safety is the primary concern in all pharmaceutical operations, and this verification step is an essential safeguard in preventing medication mix-ups, particularly in busy pharmacy settings.

Q4. Answer: C
Explanation: Verifying the completeness and legibility of the prescription is the technician's first step in ensuring accuracy. This includes checking the patient's information, medication name, strength, and dosage instructions. A clear, complete prescription helps avoid errors in data entry and ensures the pharmacist can verify it properly. This step is fundamental in maintaining accurate pharmacy operations and ensuring patient safety before dispensing.

Q5. Answer: A
Explanation: Recommending an over-the-counter product involves clinical judgment, which is outside the technician's scope. Technicians are not authorized to assess symptoms or make therapeutic recommendations. Only a pharmacist has the clinical expertise to evaluate a patient's condition and suggest appropriate treatment. Technicians can assist by providing product information or ensuring availability, but they cannot make clinical decisions for patients.

Q6. Answer: B
Explanation: Maintaining accurate inventory records ensures that medications are available when needed and prevents shortages or overstocking. This responsibility helps reduce the risk of medication errors, expired drugs, and unnecessary costs. Proper inventory management supports pharmacy operations by ensuring the right products are on hand for patient care, enhancing workflow, and ensuring that medications are safe to use within their designated expiration periods.

Q7. Answer: C
Explanation: Counting, pouring, and packaging medications are essential tasks performed by pharmacy technicians. These duties involve preparing medications as per prescription orders before the pharmacist conducts a final check. The technician's role ensures that medications are ready for verification, ensuring smooth workflow and reducing wait times for patients. This task does not involve clinical decision-making and is within the technician's scope.

Q8. Answer: B
Explanation: Protecting patient confidentiality is an essential ethical duty for pharmacy technicians. They must safeguard all sensitive patient information, following HIPAA regulations, and ensure it is shared only with authorized personnel. Maintaining confidentiality ensures trust, compliance with privacy laws, and demonstrates professionalism within the pharmacy. Discussing medical conditions in public or altering prescriptions goes against ethical standards and legal requirements.

Q9. Answer: D
Explanation: Any request involving a dosage change requires clinical evaluation and decision-making, which is beyond the technician's scope of practice. The technician must immediately notify the pharmacist to ensure that any adjustments are properly assessed for safety and effectiveness. The pharmacist has the clinical knowledge to review and approve dosage changes, ensuring the patient receives appropriate therapy.
Q10. Answer: B
Explanation: A clean and organized workspace is crucial to prevent medication contamination, errors, or mix-ups. Technicians are responsible for ensuring that work areas are kept orderly, tools are sanitized, and medications are handled in a manner that maintains their safety and effectiveness. This practice contributes to the overall safety and efficiency of the pharmacy, supporting accurate and timely medication dispensing.
Q11. Answer: B
Explanation: When faced with unclear or illegible handwriting, the technician should consult the pharmacist for clarification. The pharmacist has the authority to contact the prescriber and verify the correct medication, ensuring the prescription is filled safely. The technician's role is to assist in ensuring accuracy, but contacting the prescriber directly is beyond the technician's scope and could compromise patient safety.
Q12. Answer: B
Explanation: Sharing updates about prescription issues ensures effective teamwork and coordination. Clear communication helps prevent mistakes, delays, or misunderstandings in pharmacy workflow. Team members rely on one another for accurate information, and maintaining open lines of communication promotes patient safety, operational efficiency, and a supportive work environment. Effective teamwork is essential to delivering quality healthcare in a busy pharmacy setting.
Q13. Answer: A
Explanation: Confirming expiration dates ensures that the medications dispensed are safe and effective. Expired drugs may lose potency or become unsafe, leading to treatment failure or harm. Technicians must verify the expiration dates of medications during inventory checks, dispensing, and storage to comply with safety standards and maintain patient health and regulatory compliance. This ensures that patients receive the intended therapeutic benefit.
Q14. Answer: B
Explanation: Entering prescription data accurately is a critical responsibility that requires great attention to detail. Even a small mistake can result in the wrong medication being dispensed, which could endanger the patient's health. Technicians must ensure that all prescription information is transcribed correctly, allowing the pharmacist to verify it before dispensing. Precision in data entry is essential to maintaining pharmacy safety and efficiency.
Q15. Answer: C
Explanation: Wearing identification badges helps to identify pharmacy staff and their respective roles clearly to patients and colleagues. It ensures professional transparency and accountability, helping patients understand who is assisting them. The badge also fosters a sense of trust, making it easier to verify the credentials of those involved in the dispensing process. It complies with workplace policies and regulatory standards for safety and professionalism.
Q16. Answer: A
Explanation: Verifying the patient's identification is essential when dealing with controlled substances to ensure they are receiving the prescribed medication. This step helps prevent fraud, abuse, or diversion of drugs. The technician's responsibility is to follow proper procedures, alert the pharmacist of any concerns, and ensure that all legal requirements are met before processing the prescription.
Q17. Answer: B

Explanation: The technician must inform the patient that identification is required to complete the prescription pickup. This policy ensures that medications are dispensed to the correct person, complying with safety regulations. The pharmacist can review the situation if needed, but the technician is responsible for enforcing identification protocols to prevent potential errors and safeguard the patient's health.

Q18. Answer: C

Explanation: The technician should immediately inform the pharmacist about any allergy warnings on the prescription. The pharmacist is responsible for assessing the significance of the warning and determining whether it affects the medication choice. The technician's role is to support the pharmacist in ensuring that patients are not put at risk due to allergies or contraindications in the prescribed medications.

Q19. Answer: A

Explanation: Pediatric prescriptions often require adjusted dosages based on the child's weight or age. The technician must ensure the dosage is appropriate and verify the details with the pharmacist to ensure the accuracy of the prescription before dispensing. This precaution prevents medication errors, ensuring the child receives the correct amount for safe and effective treatment.

Q20. Answer: C

Explanation: Stock rotation is crucial in pharmacy practice to prevent expired medications from being dispensed. Technicians must place new stock behind existing stock, ensuring that older medications are used first. This process helps maintain inventory accuracy, reduces waste, and ensures that patients receive safe, effective medications within their expiration dates. Proper stock management is vital for efficient pharmacy operations.

Q21. Answer: D

Explanation: In the case of a drug recall, the technician is responsible for removing affected products from the pharmacy shelf and notifying the pharmacist immediately. The pharmacist will then handle further actions, such as notifying patients, arranging returns, or disposing of the recalled drugs. The technician's role ensures the recall process is carried out quickly and safely, minimizing patient risk.

Q22. Answer: C

Explanation: If a patient expresses concerns about a medication, the technician should inform the pharmacist, who can address the patient's concerns, provide counseling, or discuss possible alternatives. Technicians do not have the authority to change or recommend medications independently. Addressing patient concerns is a collaborative process, with the pharmacist providing expert guidance on medication safety and efficacy.

Q23. Answer: A

Explanation: If a prescription contains a known allergen, the technician should notify the pharmacist immediately. The pharmacist will assess the situation, check for alternatives, and decide whether a substitution or additional steps are necessary. The technician should not make changes to prescriptions or override allergy warnings without professional guidance. Ensuring patient safety is the top priority.

Q24. Answer: B

Explanation: The technician should immediately verify any discrepancies or unusual dosage forms with the pharmacist. This ensures the correct medication is dispensed as per the doctor's instructions. Dosage forms must align with the prescription details, and any confusion should be addressed before processing to ensure patient safety and regulatory compliance.

Q25. Answer: C

Explanation: Pharmacy technicians should always follow the pharmacist's instructions when providing medication counseling. Technicians are not authorized to offer medical advice or discuss side effects in depth. The pharmacist, as the healthcare professional, is responsible for counseling patients on side effects and drug interactions. Technicians assist in ensuring that patients understand proper usage by supporting the pharmacist's guidance.

Q26. Answer: C

Explanation: Pharmacy technicians are responsible for preparing medications, including counting, measuring, and labeling prescriptions, for pharmacist review. They do not make clinical decisions, such as choosing dosages or performing assessments. Technicians assist in ensuring that prescriptions are prepared accurately and in compliance with safety standards before the pharmacist verifies and dispenses them. This ensures workflow efficiency and patient safety.

Q27. Answer: B

Explanation: Double-checking medication labels before dispensing is crucial to patient safety. This helps prevent dispensing errors, such as incorrect medication or dosage. Pharmacy technicians must verify that the information matches the prescription details and that labels are clear and legible. Ensuring accuracy before final verification by the pharmacist minimizes the risk of harm to the patient and ensures compliance with safety protocols.

Q28. Answer: B

Explanation: If a medication error occurs, the technician must inform the pharmacist immediately so they can take corrective action. Documenting the error ensures proper reporting and helps improve future pharmacy practices. The pharmacist will assess the situation, inform the patient if necessary, and determine the next steps to correct the mistake. Transparency and quick action are essential to patient safety and regulatory compliance.

Q29. Answer: A

Explanation: Verifying a patient's allergy information is critical to avoiding potentially harmful interactions between the patient's allergies and the medications prescribed. Pharmacy technicians should always check patient records for allergies before dispensing any medications. This precaution helps prevent adverse reactions that could harm the patient, ensuring safe and effective treatment. It is an essential part of patient care and safety protocols in the pharmacy.

Q30. Answer: B

Explanation: When handling controlled substances, the technician's first action is to verify the patient's identity and ensure compliance with all regulatory requirements, such as checking ID and reviewing the prescription for accuracy. Controlled substances are subject to stricter legal regulations to prevent misuse or diversion. The technician must follow all procedures carefully, reporting any discrepancies or concerns to the pharmacist for further action.

Q31. Answer: B

Explanation: Staying current with drug formulations and dosages ensures that pharmacy technicians can prepare and dispense medications accurately. This knowledge helps prevent medication errors, ensuring that patients receive the correct drug in the correct form and dosage. It is essential for technicians to be familiar with new and existing medications to support pharmacists in providing safe and effective patient care.

Q32. Answer: B

Explanation: If a patient requests a medication not on the pharmacy's formulary, the technician should suggest an alternative, if available, and consult the pharmacist. The pharmacist can then assess whether a suitable substitution is available or work with the patient's physician to fulfill the prescription. The technician should not independently dispense or refuse without consulting the pharmacist, as they lack the authority to make clinical decisions.

Q33. Answer: C

Explanation: The primary duty of pharmacy technicians in sterile compounding is to prepare medications while maintaining strict aseptic technique. This includes accurately measuring ingredients, mixing medications, and ensuring that the environment remains sterile to prevent contamination. Technicians support the pharmacist's role by preparing compounds safely and following regulatory guidelines, ensuring patient safety and adherence to proper pharmaceutical standards.

Q34. Answer: D

Explanation: Pharmacy technicians can prevent medication errors by adhering to established procedures, verifying prescription information, and double-checking medication orders before dispensing. This includes confirming dosage, drug form, and patient details. By following these protocols, technicians ensure that medications are accurately prepared and dispensed, minimizing the risk of errors. Their attention to detail supports the pharmacist in maintaining patient safety and compliance with pharmacy regulations.

Q35. Answer: C

Explanation: When a discrepancy in dosage occurs, the technician should consult the pharmacist immediately. The pharmacist will review the prescription for accuracy and make the necessary clinical decisions. Technicians are not authorized to alter prescription details. Consulting the pharmacist ensures that the patient receives the correct medication in the appropriate dosage and prevents potential safety issues.

Q36. Answer: B

Explanation: Patient counseling is an essential service provided by pharmacists, where patients are given detailed information about their prescribed medications. This includes instructions on how to use the medication, potential side effects, and what to do if they experience any issues. Counseling ensures that patients understand their treatment plan, leading to better medication adherence and improved health outcomes. Pharmacy technicians assist by preparing the medications for counseling.

Q37. Answer: B

Explanation: Look-alike, sound-alike drugs are a significant risk factor for medication errors, as they can be easily confused due to similar names or appearances. Pharmacy technicians should be vigilant and verify drug names, ensuring the correct medication is dispensed. Being aware of these similarities helps reduce the risk of dispensing the wrong drug, promoting patient safety and accuracy in pharmacy practice.

Q38. Answer: B

Explanation: Discussing patient prescriptions in private with the pharmacist is permissible and is required to ensure confidentiality. HIPAA regulations mandate that all patient information remains confidential and only accessible to authorized individuals in secure settings. Sharing personal or medical information in public or with unauthorized persons violates patient privacy and could result in legal consequences for the pharmacy and the technician.

Q39. Answer: A

Explanation: Pharmacy technicians should always request clarification from a pharmacist if they are unsure about any aspect of a prescription, such as the medication's name, dosage, or instructions. It is essential to ensure the prescription is accurate before dispensing, as mistakes could lead to patient harm. Pharmacists are responsible for providing guidance on any issues or questions about prescriptions, maintaining patient safety and regulatory compliance.

Q40. Answer: C

Explanation: Before dispensing controlled substances, pharmacy technicians must verify the patient's ID and ensure that the prescription is valid. This includes checking for proper authorization, prescription quantity limits, and documentation required for controlled substances. Strict regulatory controls are in place for controlled medications to prevent abuse and misuse, and technicians must follow these protocols carefully to ensure compliance and patient safety.

Q41. Answer: D

Explanation: Pharmacy technicians assist with sterile compounding by preparing medications according to the pharmacist's instructions while maintaining aseptic techniques. This ensures that compounded medications are safe, effective, and free from contamination. Technicians play a key role in preparing sterile products but must always follow safety and regulatory guidelines, under the direct supervision of a pharmacist, to ensure the quality of the final product.

Q42. Answer: C

Explanation: Dispensing medication without a valid prescription is a serious ethical and legal violation. Pharmacy technicians must always ensure that prescriptions are valid, accurate, and authorized before dispensing medications. Working within the scope of practice and adhering to legal regulations is critical to maintaining patient safety, compliance with pharmacy laws, and ethical standards. Violating these principles can lead to legal consequences and harm to patients.

Q43. Answer: B

Explanation: Staying informed about new drug developments ensures pharmacy technicians can properly handle and dispense medications. This includes understanding new formulations, dosages, and administration routes. Staying updated helps prevent errors and supports the pharmacist in making informed decisions about patient care. It also ensures that the pharmacy complies with industry standards and regulations for safe medication management.

Q44. Answer: B

Explanation: If a pharmacy technician is uncertain about a prescription, they must consult the pharmacist for clarification. The pharmacist has the clinical expertise to verify the medication and provide guidance on correct dispensing. Technicians are responsible for accurately preparing medications but must rely on the pharmacist's expertise to ensure the prescription is filled safely, especially in uncertain situations or with unfamiliar drugs.

Q45. Answer: D

Explanation: When receiving a prescription for a controlled substance, the technician must verify the patient's identity and ensure the prescription is complete. This includes checking for correct patient details, physician authorization, and necessary documentation as required by law. Controlled substances are highly regulated, and thorough verification helps ensure compliance with legal requirements and prevents the misuse or diversion of medications.

Q46. Answer: A

Explanation: The National Drug Code uniquely identifies the manufacturer, strength, and dosage form of a medication. Verifying the NDC ensures the exact product prescribed is dispensed, reducing the risk of selection errors.

Q47. Answer: B

Explanation: Dividing the prescribed dose (250 mg) by the available tablet strength (125 mg) equals 2 tablets. Accurate calculations ensure the patient receives the intended therapeutic dose.

Q48. Answer: B

Explanation: Comparing the stock bottle to the prescription label confirms the correct medication and strength are selected. This verification step is critical in preventing dispensing errors.

Q49. Answer: C

Explanation: A concentration of 100 mg per 5 mL means that each 5 mL dose contains 100 mg. Understanding concentration ensures correct dose preparation and administration.

Q50. Answer: B

Explanation: Medications beyond their expiration date may lose potency or stability. Checking expiration dates ensures safety, effectiveness, and compliance with pharmacy standards.

Q51. Answer: B

Explanation: The pharmacy technician must check the patient's valid photo ID when dispensing controlled substances. This ensures the person receiving the medication is indeed the prescribed individual. Compliance with this verification is essential in preventing fraud and misuse of controlled substances. In some states, the PDMP is also checked, but the photo ID is the primary document for identity verification before dispensing.

Q52. Answer: B

Explanation: Pharmacy technicians must ensure that medications are stocked and rotated based on expiration dates. This is essential for preventing the dispensing of expired medications, which could pose risks to patient health. Proper inventory management helps maintain medication quality, minimize waste, and ensure that patients receive the correct and safe medications. It also supports overall pharmacy efficiency and regulatory compliance.

Q53. Answer: C

Explanation: The drug's expiration date must always be included on the medication label. This is a critical safety feature, ensuring that patients only receive effective medications that are still within their potency and safety limits. It also helps comply with regulatory standards and prevents dispensing expired medications, which could lose their therapeutic effectiveness or cause adverse effects.

Q54. Answer: B

Explanation: Misbranding occurs when a medication is labeled incorrectly, such as providing incorrect dosage instructions or failing to include important safety information. This could lead to medication errors and patient harm. Proper labeling is a regulatory requirement, and technicians must ensure that all information, including dosage and directions, is correct before the medication is dispensed. Misbranding can lead to legal consequences and jeopardize patient safety.

Q55. Answer: A

Explanation: If a patient is unable to understand medication instructions, the pharmacy technician should refer them to the pharmacist for counseling. The pharmacist can provide detailed explanations about the medication, its purpose, and its proper usage. Technicians are not authorized to provide detailed clinical advice, but they play a key role in ensuring patients understand their treatment with the pharmacist's help.

Q56. Answer: B

Explanation: Talking to a colleague about a patient's medical history, unless that colleague is involved in patient care, is a violation of patient confidentiality. Pharmacy technicians must maintain strict confidentiality in all patient interactions, sharing information only with authorized personnel involved in the patient's care. Confidentiality is a legal and ethical obligation, ensuring trust and compliance with healthcare privacy laws such as HIPAA.

Q57. Answer: D

Explanation: Pharmacy technicians should understand drug interactions to assist the pharmacist in identifying and preventing harmful interactions. Technicians may not be involved in clinical decision-making but must be aware of potential interactions to flag concerns for the pharmacist's review. This knowledge helps maintain patient safety and ensures that medications are prescribed and dispensed in a way that minimizes adverse effects or treatment failure.

Q58. Answer: B

Explanation: A black box warning indicates that a medication carries significant risk for severe side effects. Pharmacy technicians must always alert the pharmacist when processing such prescriptions. The pharmacist will discuss the warning with the patient and ensure they are informed of the potential risks. Technicians cannot provide counseling but can help facilitate the pharmacist's review and ensure the patient understands the safety precautions.

Q59. Answer: C

Explanation: If a medication is out of stock, the technician should notify the pharmacist immediately. The pharmacist can assess whether there is an appropriate alternative or determine when the medication will be available. Technicians should not make decisions regarding substitutions without consulting the pharmacist, as they lack the clinical knowledge to make such determinations. This ensures that the patient receives the most suitable medication.

Q60. Answer: B

Explanation: If a pharmacy technician receives expired medication, it should be returned to the supplier immediately for replacement. Dispensing expired medications is against regulatory guidelines and could endanger patient health. Technicians must follow proper procedures for handling expired stock to maintain patient safety and ensure compliance with pharmacy regulations. Proper disposal or return of expired medications is crucial to prevent legal or safety violations.

Q61. Answer: C

Explanation: Drug reference materials, such as drug guides or databases, help pharmacy technicians accurately prepare and label medications with the correct details, including dosage, usage, and potential interactions. Knowing how to use these resources ensures that technicians provide safe and effective medications to patients. While technicians cannot offer clinical advice, using references helps them support pharmacists and ensure accurate medication dispensing.

Q62. Answer: A

Explanation: If a pharmacy technician notices a medication error while labeling or preparing the prescription, they must notify the pharmacist immediately. This prevents the medication from being dispensed incorrectly and ensures patient safety. The pharmacist will review the error and take appropriate action, such as correcting the prescription or contacting the patient. Early detection and reporting of errors are crucial for preventing harm.

Q63. Answer: B

Explanation: Medications that require refrigeration should be stored in a designated refrigerator with appropriate temperature control. This ensures that they remain effective and safe to use. The technician is responsible for regularly checking the refrigerator's temperature and making sure it is within the required range. Proper storage is crucial for maintaining medication potency and adhering to regulatory standards for pharmaceutical care.

Q64. Answer: B

Explanation: Pharmacy technicians must follow strict guidelines for handling, storing, and disposing of hazardous drugs. This includes wearing protective equipment, such as gloves and gowns, and using special containment systems. Proper handling minimizes the risk of exposure and ensures that the drugs are safely dispensed or disposed of in accordance with regulations. The technician's role is vital in maintaining a safe environment in the pharmacy.

Q65. Answer: D

Explanation: The technician must follow the manufacturer's instructions for the correct solvent and method of reconstitution. Using the wrong solvent or incorrect procedure could affect the medication's potency, safety, and effectiveness. The pharmacist typically verifies these details before the technician prepares the medication, ensuring that the drug is correctly reconstituted according to specifications. Proper reconstitution is critical to maintaining the drug's therapeutic efficacy.

Q66. Answer: C

Explanation: If a medication is damaged, the technician should immediately notify the pharmacist and place it in the designated area for damaged goods. This ensures that the medication is properly assessed for potential loss of potency or contamination. The pharmacist will decide the next steps, whether it be returning it to the supplier or disposing of it safely. Damaged medications must not be dispensed.

Q67. Answer: C

Explanation: If a prescription specifies "no refills," the pharmacy technician must process the prescription exactly as written. Adding refills would be a violation of pharmacy practice and could lead to legal and ethical issues. The technician should ensure that the medication is dispensed accurately, and if further refills are needed, the patient must contact their prescribing healthcare provider for a new prescription.

Q68. Answer: B

Explanation: Sharing patient records with unauthorized individuals is a direct violation of privacy laws such as HIPAA. Pharmacy technicians must safeguard patient information and ensure it is only shared with authorized individuals involved in the patient's care. Patient confidentiality is a fundamental ethical and legal responsibility. Any breach could result in legal consequences, compromise patient trust, and violate healthcare regulations.

Q69. Answer: B

Explanation: Upon noticing a medication recall, the pharmacy technician must immediately inform the pharmacist and remove the affected product from stock. This is critical for patient safety, as recalled medications may be harmful or ineffective. The pharmacist will guide the next steps, such as contacting patients or arranging for the return of the recalled product. Quick action helps protect patients and maintain pharmacy integrity.

Q70. Answer: C

Explanation: Verifying the medication's correct dosage form and ensuring that the label matches the prescription is a primary responsibility of pharmacy technicians. This step is critical to ensure the patient receives the correct medication and dosage. Technicians must accurately prepare and label medications under the supervision of a pharmacist. They do not adjust dosages or provide clinical counseling, which is outside their scope.

Q71. Answer: B

Explanation: If a pharmacy technician finds a medication error during the dispensing process, they should immediately report the error to the pharmacist and halt the dispensing process. The pharmacist will assess the situation and determine the necessary steps to correct the error. Ensuring medication accuracy is vital to patient safety, and reporting the error helps prevent dispensing incorrect medication, protecting both the patient and the pharmacy.

Q72. Answer: A

Explanation: Pediatric dosages often depend on the child's weight to ensure that the medication is administered safely and effectively. Verifying the child's weight before dispensing ensures that the prescribed dosage is appropriate for the patient's size and prevents the risk of underdose or overdose. This is a critical step in safeguarding pediatric patients, as their bodies respond differently to medications compared to adults.

Q73. Answer: C

Explanation: If a pharmacy technician notices an issue with a narcotic prescription, they must immediately alert the pharmacist. Narcotics are highly regulated, and any discrepancies or concerns about the prescription must be addressed before dispensing. The pharmacist will verify the prescription's validity, check for any red flags, and ensure that it complies with legal and safety standards. The technician must not process the prescription without the pharmacist's approval.

Q74. Answer: C

Explanation: Medications with controlled access, such as narcotics, must be stored securely in locked cabinets or safes. Access should be restricted to authorized personnel, and only when necessary for dispensing. Pharmacy technicians must follow strict protocols for handling, storing, and tracking these medications to prevent misuse, diversion, or theft. Proper documentation of inventory and dispensing is essential to ensure compliance with regulatory standards and maintain patient safety.

Q75. Answer: B

Explanation: If a pharmacy technician is unsure about a specific drug interaction, they should consult a drug reference or immediately ask the pharmacist for guidance. Pharmacists are the clinical experts responsible for ensuring that prescribed drugs do not interact in harmful ways. Technicians must rely on the pharmacist's expertise and resources to resolve any concerns and ensure patient safety before dispensing the medication.

Q76. Answer: B

Explanation: Pharmacy technicians must ensure medications requiring special storage, like refrigeration, are stored properly in controlled environments to maintain their potency and safety. Proper storage ensures that the medication remains effective and within regulatory guidelines. Storing medications correctly prevents degradation and ensures that patients receive safe and effective treatments. Regular temperature checks and adherence to storage guidelines are crucial parts of the technician's role.

Q77. Answer: C

Explanation: High-risk medications, such as those with narrow therapeutic windows or complex dosing, require extra attention. The pharmacy technician should always verify the prescription with the pharmacist and double-check the dosage, ensuring that the medication is dispensed safely. Extra verification helps minimize the risk of errors and ensures that the medication will be effective and safe for the patient's specific needs.

Q78. Answer: B

Explanation: When dispensing medication in a blister pack, the pharmacy technician must verify that the medication matches the prescription and that each blister contains the correct dose. This ensures the patient receives the correct medication and dosage, as blister packs are pre-packaged for convenience and safety. Technicians must ensure that there are no discrepancies and that all medication is dispensed according to the prescription.

Q79. Answer: D

Explanation: Pharmacy technicians assist in medication therapy management (MTM) by gathering and reviewing a patient's medication history and providing relevant information to the pharmacist. Technicians do not independently adjust treatment regimens or conduct clinical assessments, which are the responsibilities of pharmacists. MTM is a collaborative process where the pharmacist uses the technician's gathered information to optimize the patient's medication regimen, improving therapeutic outcomes.

Q80. Answer: B

Explanation: The pharmacy technician should immediately alert the pharmacist to the patient's known penicillin allergy. The pharmacist will assess the prescription, check for any possible cross-reactivity, and determine if a suitable alternative medication should be provided. The technician cannot change or alter medications independently, and ignoring allergy warnings could result in severe adverse reactions. Communication with the pharmacist ensures patient safety.

Q81. Answer: B

Explanation: When handling hazardous medications, pharmacy technicians must wear appropriate personal protective equipment (PPE), including gloves, gowns, and face shields or masks. This protects them from potential exposure to harmful substances that can cause serious health risks. PPE is essential to prevent contamination and ensure the safety of both the technician and other personnel. Safe handling practices also comply with regulatory guidelines for hazardous drug management.

Q82. Answer: B

Explanation: When a medication shortage occurs, the pharmacy technician should immediately inform the pharmacist and check for any available alternatives or substitutions. The pharmacist will review the situation and, if necessary, contact the prescribing healthcare provider to discuss treatment options with the patient. The technician plays an important role in ensuring that patients receive the best available medication in a timely and safe manner.

Q83. Answer: C

Explanation: If a prescription is missing a doctor's signature, the pharmacy technician must immediately inform the pharmacist and refrain from dispensing the medication. Prescriptions that lack the proper authorization are invalid, and dispensing such medications could violate legal and regulatory guidelines. The pharmacist will contact the healthcare provider to resolve the issue and ensure that the prescription is properly signed before processing.

Q84. Answer: A

Explanation: Following proper hand hygiene is critical to preventing medication contamination and ensuring safety. Pharmacy technicians must wash their hands regularly and use hand sanitizers to reduce the risk of spreading germs or contaminating medications, which could harm patients. Cleanliness is essential for maintaining a sterile environment and ensuring that all medications are dispensed in accordance with pharmaceutical safety standards. Proper hygiene supports overall patient health and safety.

Q85. Answer: D

Explanation: Controlled substances require strict regulation, and prescriptions for them should be verified with a pharmacist, even if presented after hours. The technician must ensure compliance with state and federal laws, including ensuring the prescription is valid. The pharmacist must review the prescription for accuracy and legality before dispensing. Regulations may require special documentation or additional steps, and the technician must follow these procedures carefully to ensure compliance.

Q86. Answer: C

Explanation: Pharmacy technicians should consult the pharmacist if they notice or are unsure about a potential drug-drug interaction. Since technicians are not qualified to interpret interactions independently, they must rely on the pharmacist's expertise to assess the safety of combinations of medications. The pharmacist will evaluate the potential interactions and provide guidance to ensure that the patient receives the correct treatment without adverse effects.

Q87. Answer: B

Explanation: To maintain the security of medications, pharmacy technicians must lock up controlled substances and other high-risk medications in designated secure areas when not in use. This practice prevents theft, misuse, and accidental access. Ensuring that medications are kept in secure areas is vital for maintaining regulatory compliance and protecting both patients and the pharmacy from potential liabilities related to medication diversion or loss.

Q88. Answer: B

Explanation: If a mistake is made during medication preparation, the technician should immediately inform the pharmacist and correct the mistake. The pharmacist will oversee the correction process and ensure that the medication is dispensed safely. Addressing mistakes quickly ensures that patient safety is not compromised and that the pharmacy complies with regulatory standards for safe dispensing practices. Timely error correction prevents further issues.

Q89. Answer: D

Explanation: The pharmacist is responsible for ensuring that special handling instructions are communicated to the patient. While pharmacy technicians may assist in preparing the medication and labeling it, they do not provide clinical counseling. The pharmacist will explain the handling instructions, such as refrigeration or administration guidelines, and ensure the patient understands how to use the medication safely. This role is critical to medication adherence and patient safety.

Q90. Answer: B

Explanation: The pharmacy technician must check for potential drug interactions and verify that the dosages are correct when processing a prescription for a patient with multiple medications. Although the technician is not responsible for clinical decision-making, they must flag any concerns for the pharmacist's review. Ensuring that medications are compatible and appropriately dosed helps prevent adverse reactions and ensures that the patient receives safe, effective therapy.

Q91. Answer: C

Explanation: The DEA enforces laws related to controlled substances under the Controlled Substances Act. It oversees drug scheduling, registration, and recordkeeping to prevent misuse and diversion. While the FDA governs drug safety and efficacy, the DEA's primary focus is preventing illegal distribution and ensuring controlled substances are used properly in medical and research settings. The CDC and FTC have unrelated roles in public health and consumer protection respectively.

Q92. Answer: B

Explanation: The CSA classifies drugs into Schedules I–V based on their accepted medical use and potential for abuse or dependency. Schedule I drugs have no accepted medical use and high abuse risk, while Schedule V drugs have limited abuse potential. This classification system ensures appropriate prescribing, handling, and legal penalties. Cost, brand status, or dosage form are unrelated to scheduling decisions, which are made primarily on safety and abuse data.

Q93. Answer: A

Explanation: DEA Form 222 is used for the purchase and transfer of Schedule II controlled substances between registrants. It documents the exact drug, strength, quantity, and recipient to ensure traceability and prevent diversion. Form 41 covers destruction of controlled substances, Form 106 reports theft or loss, and Form 224 is for initial DEA registration. Thus, only Form 222 is valid for legally ordering Schedule II substances under DEA regulations.

Q94. Answer: C

Explanation: Upon discovering loss or theft of controlled substances, the pharmacist-in-charge must be notified, and a DEA Form 106 must be completed to report the incident to the DEA. This form documents drug name, quantity, and circumstances. Form 41 is used only for drug destruction, while the FDA has no jurisdiction in this case. Prompt reporting ensures compliance and helps identify diversion sources for security and accountability.

Q95. Answer: D

Explanation: Federal law strictly prohibits refills for Schedule II controlled substances. Each prescription requires a new written or electronic order from a prescriber. This restriction helps control abuse and diversion of high-risk medications such as opioids and stimulants. In contrast, Schedules III–V allow limited refills within specific time frames. Attempting to refill a Schedule II prescription violates DEA regulations and may result in legal and professional penalties.

Q96. Answer: B

Explanation: Schedule III drugs have accepted medical uses but possess a moderate to low potential for physical or psychological dependence. Examples include certain combination products containing limited quantities of narcotics. These medications balance therapeutic benefit with risk management under DEA oversight. Schedule I substances have no accepted medical use, while Schedules IV and V have progressively lower abuse potential and dependency risks.

Q97. Answer: B

Explanation: Federal regulations mandate that DEA 222 forms and controlled substance records be kept for at least two years from the date of the last entry. These records must be readily retrievable for inspection by the DEA or state boards. Maintaining accurate documentation ensures accountability and traceability of controlled substances. Shorter retention violates federal law, while longer retention, though permissible, exceeds the required compliance period.

Q98. Answer: D

Explanation: Schedule III and IV drugs can be refilled up to five times within six months from the prescription date, per federal law. Beyond this limit, a new prescription is required. This regulation helps monitor patient use and prevents misuse of potentially addictive medications such as benzodiazepines. Schedules I and II cannot be refilled, and Schedules V drugs may be refilled more flexibly based on state laws.

Q99. Answer: B

Explanation: The Poison Prevention Packaging Act (PPPA) mandates child-resistant containers for most prescription and over-the-counter medications to prevent accidental poisoning. It is enforced by the Consumer Product Safety Commission (CPSC). Certain exceptions apply for specific medications or patient requests. The CSA governs controlled substances, while the FD&C Act ensures drug safety and labeling. The PPPA specifically targets physical packaging safety to protect children from accidental ingestion.

Q100. Answer: C

Explanation: Hydrocodone, including combination products, is classified as a Schedule II controlled substance due to its high abuse potential and potential for severe dependence. Alprazolam and diazepam are Schedule IV benzodiazepines, indicating lower risk. Pregabalin is Schedule V, with minimal abuse potential. Understanding these classifications ensures correct storage, dispensing, and documentation, reducing legal risk and promoting patient safety within pharmacy practice.

Questions (101-200)

Q101. Which element must be present on a valid controlled substance prescription to verify the prescriber's authority?

A. Prescriber signature and DEA number

B. Pharmacy initials only

C. Patient insurance card copy

D. Manufacturer lot number

Q102. Under HIPAA, which of the following is considered Protected Health Information (PHI)?

A. Patient name and diagnosis

B. Pharmacy inventory counts

C. Manufacturer NDC codes

D. Drug expiration dates

Q103. Which federal law requires pharmacies to offer counseling to Medicaid patients about their medications?

A. Controlled Substances Act

B. Poison Prevention Packaging Act

C. Omnibus Budget Reconciliation Act (OBRA) 1990

D. Food, Drug, and Cosmetic Act

Q104. What is the primary purpose of the Drug Supply Chain Security Act (DSCSA)?

A. Establish track-and-trace systems to protect the drug supply

B. Mandate child-resistant packaging

C. Restrict OTC medication sales

D. Create formularies for hospitals

Q105. Which inventory control practice is specifically required for Schedule II controlled substances?

A. Perpetual inventory with accurate count

B. Annual physical count only

C. No documentation required

D. Store with OTC stock

Q106. When transferring a Schedule III–V prescription between pharmacies, which statement is true under federal law?

A. There is no limit on transfers for Schedules III–V

B. A controlled prescription may be transferred only once between pharmacies

C. Transfers for controlled substances are prohibited

D. Transfers require DEA Form 222

Q107. Which federal regulation addresses safe handling and disposal of hazardous drugs in healthcare settings?

A. USP <800>

B. Controlled Substances Act

C. HIPAA

D. Poison Prevention Packaging Act

Q108. Which requirement applies when a pharmacy receives a forged prescription for a controlled substance?

A. Refuse to fill and notify the pharmacist and law enforcement

B. Fill the prescription to avoid patient harm

C. Alter the prescriber name to the on-duty physician

D. Fax it to another pharmacy for verification

Q109. Which action is required if a controlled substance inventory shows a discrepancy suggesting diversion?
A. Return stock to the wholesaler without notice
B. Ignore and continue dispensing
C. Immediately destroy remaining stock without documentation
D. Conduct an internal investigation, notify the pharmacist-in-charge, and report to DEA if necessary
Q110. Under federal law, which practitioner identifier must be used when billing Medicare Part D prescriptions?
A. National Provider Identifier (NPI)
B. Social Security number
C. Employee badge number
D. State pharmacy license number
Q111. Which law requires pharmacies to maintain records of prescription drug returns and destructions?
A. Controlled Substances Act (CSA) and DEA regulations
B. HIPAA
C. Poison Prevention Packaging Act
D. Fair Labor Standards Act
Q112. What is required on a prescription label for a controlled substance when dispensing to a patient?
A. Only drug name and quantity
B. Patient name, drug name and strength, directions, prescriber name, and pharmacy information
C. Manufacturer contact info only
D. Insurance plan and BIN number
Q113. Under HIPAA, when may a pharmacy disclose PHI without patient authorization?
A. For treatment, payment, or healthcare operations
B. For marketing unrelated products
C. To post patient lists publicly
D. To release patient SSNs to employers
Q114. Which document is used to report significant adverse events to the FDA?
A. MedWatch Form 3500
B. DEA Form 222
C. CMS-1500
D. OSHA Form 300
Q115. Which regulation outlines requirements for packaging to prevent child access to medications?
A. Drug Supply Chain Security Act
B. HIPAA Privacy Rule
C. Poison Prevention Packaging Act (PPPA)
D. OSHA Hazard Communication Standard
Q116. What is the main function of the Controlled Substances Act (CSA)?
A. Regulate the safety of over-the-counter medications
B. Control the manufacture and distribution of potentially addictive drugs
C. Establish labeling requirements for dietary supplements
D. Oversee food safety and inspections
Q117. A DEA Form 41 must be used for which pharmacy activity?
A. Destruction of expired controlled substances
B. Ordering Schedule II medications
C. Reporting theft or loss
D. Registering a new pharmacy

Q118. Which of the following is true about DEA registration renewal for pharmacies?
A. Renewal occurs every year
B. Renewal occurs every three years
C. Renewal occurs every five years
D. No renewal is necessary
Q119. How should expired Schedule II medications be disposed of?
A. Through DEA-authorized reverse distributors
B. By returning them to patients
C. By flushing them down the drain
D. By throwing them in regular trash
Q120. The Combat Methamphetamine Epidemic Act restricts the sale of which substances?
A. Pseudoephedrine and ephedrine
B. Ibuprofen and acetaminophen
C. Loratadine and cetirizine
D. Diphenhydramine and chlorpheniramine
Q121. What is the maximum amount of pseudoephedrine a customer may purchase in one day under federal law?
A. 7.5 grams
B. 9 grams
C. 5 grams
D. 3.6 grams
Q122. When a prescriber issues an emergency oral prescription for a Schedule II drug, the pharmacy must receive a written or electronic prescription within how many days?
A. 3 days
B. 7 days
C. 10 days
D. 14 days
Q123. Which of the following actions would violate DEA storage requirements for controlled substances?
A. Keeping Schedule II drugs in an unlocked cabinet
B. Using a double-locked cabinet
C. Storing Schedule III–V drugs with general inventory
D. Conducting daily security checks
Q124. Which law established the FDA's authority to require proof of drug efficacy before approval?
A. Kefauver-Harris Amendment
B. Durham-Humphrey Amendment
C. Controlled Substances Act
D. Drug Supply Chain Security Act
Q125. The Durham-Humphrey Amendment established which regulatory distinction?
A. Pharmacist licensing standards
B. Brand and generic labeling requirements
C. Prescription and over-the-counter drugs
D. Controlled substance schedules
Q126. Which organization assigns National Drug Codes (NDCs)?
A. Food and Drug Administration (FDA)
B. Drug Enforcement Administration (DEA)
C. Centers for Medicare and Medicaid Services (CMS)
D. United States Pharmacopeia (USP)

Q127. How often must pharmacies perform a complete inventory of all controlled substances according to federal law?

A. Every year
B. Every two years
C. Every three years
D. Every six months

Q128. Which DEA form is required to report theft or significant loss of controlled substances?

A. DEA Form 106
B. DEA Form 41
C. DEA Form 222
D. DEA Form 224

Q129. What is the primary purpose of the FDA's MedWatch program?

A. Collect and monitor reports of adverse drug events
B. Track sales of over-the-counter products
C. Regulate controlled substances
D. Manage pharmacy inspections

Q130. Under the FDA, which phase of clinical trials primarily assesses drug safety and dosage in humans?

A. Phase I
B. Phase II
C. Phase III
D. Phase IV

Q131. When must a DEA Form 222 be kept available for inspection?

A. No record retention is required
B. Only until the order is filled
C. Until the drug expires
D. Always, for at least two years after final entry

Q132. Which of the following is required before a pharmacy may dispense controlled substances electronically?

A. DEA registration and certified electronic prescription system
B. HIPAA authorization form
C. State retail permit only
D. Patient's verbal approval

Q133. Which act first required new drugs to demonstrate safety before marketing?

A. Food, Drug, and Cosmetic Act of 1938
B. Pure Food and Drug Act of 1906
C. Controlled Substances Act
D. Kefauver-Harris Amendment

Q134. Which act established the requirement for drug manufacturers to maintain truthful advertising of prescription drugs?

A. Federal Trade Commission Act
B. Food, Drug, and Cosmetic Act
C. Prescription Drug Marketing Act
D. Fair Packaging and Labeling Act

Q135. Which law mandates reporting of suspected child abuse by healthcare professionals?

A. Child Abuse Prevention and Treatment Act
B. Controlled Substances Act
C. HIPAA

D. OSHA

Q136. Which statement about Schedule V controlled substances is correct?

A. They require DEA Form 222 for ordering

B. They have the lowest abuse potential and some may be sold without a prescription

C. They cannot be refilled

D. They are only used for veterinary purposes

Q137. Who is responsible for verifying DEA registration numbers on controlled prescriptions?

A. The pharmacist

B. The pharmacy technician

C. The patient

D. The prescriber's office assistant

Q138. A prescription for alprazolam is classified under which DEA schedule?

A. Schedule II

B. Schedule III

C. Schedule IV

D. Schedule V

Q139. Which DEA form is used when a pharmacy applies for its initial registration to handle controlled substances?

A. DEA Form 224

B. DEA Form 222

C. DEA Form 106

D. DEA Form 41

Q140. Which agency enforces the Poison Prevention Packaging Act (PPPA)?

A. Consumer Product Safety Commission (CPSC)

B. Food and Drug Administration (FDA)

C. Drug Enforcement Administration (DEA)

D. Centers for Disease Control and Prevention (CDC)

Q141. What is the purpose of the Controlled Substances Ordering System (CSOS)?

A. Report medication errors to the FDA

B. Replace DEA Form 106

C. Record destruction of expired drugs

D. Allow electronic ordering of Schedule II–V drugs

Q142. Which document is required when transferring Schedule II controlled substances between DEA registrants?

A. DEA Form 222

B. DEA Form 224

C. DEA Form 41

D. DEA Form 106

Q143. How often must a pharmacy register with the DEA to dispense controlled substances?

A. Every year

B. Every three years

C. Every five years

D. One time only

Q144. Which amendment to the FD&C Act clarified prescription versus OTC labeling requirements?

A. Durham-Humphrey Amendment

B. Kefauver-Harris Amendment

C. Prescription Drug Marketing Act

D. Poison Prevention Packaging Act

Q145. What information must appear on all controlled substance prescription labels under federal law?
A. Patient name, pharmacy name/address, prescription number, date, directions, prescriber, and drug details
B. Prescriber DEA number only
C. Price and insurance information
D. Pharmacist initials only
Q146. Which agency oversees the enforcement of the Controlled Substances Act?
A. Centers for Medicare & Medicaid Services (CMS)
B. Food and Drug Administration (FDA)
C. Drug Enforcement Administration (DEA)
D. Consumer Product Safety Commission (CPSC)
Q147. In what situation may a prescriber issue multiple prescriptions for the same Schedule II drug on the same day?
A. To allow up to a 90-day total supply if each prescription has a valid future date
B. Only for hospital use
C. Never permitted under any circumstance
D. Only during drug shortages
Q148. What is the primary role of the FDA's Center for Drug Evaluation and Research (CDER)?
A. Evaluate new drug safety and effectiveness before approval
B. Regulate medical devices only
C. Monitor food labeling
D. Enforce workplace safety laws
Q149. What must be verified on a DEA registration certificate displayed in the pharmacy?
A. Drug expiration dates
B. Correct registrant name, address, and expiration date
C. Pharmacist continuing education hours
D. Employee attendance logs
Q150. Which law mandates that controlled substance records must be readily retrievable for DEA inspection?
A. Controlled Substances Act
B. HIPAA Privacy Rule
C. Poison Prevention Packaging Act
D. Prescription Drug Marketing Act
Q151. A prescriber's DEA number begins with "X." What does this indicate?
A. Authorized to prescribe buprenorphine for opioid dependence
B. Authorized to dispense Schedule I substances
C. Employed by the DEA
D. Limited to veterinary practice
Q152. How should controlled substances be stored in institutional settings like hospitals?
A. In unlocked patient drawers
B. On open shelves near nursing stations
C. With non-controlled stock for convenience
D. In a locked, substantially constructed cabinet with limited access
Q153. When a controlled substance is dispensed, which of the following must be documented immediately?
A. Date, quantity dispensed, and initials of the pharmacist
B. Patient's insurance number
C. Prescriber's state license expiration

D. Wholesaler contact information

Q154. What type of notice must accompany transferred controlled substances during reverse distribution?

A. DEA Form 222 or electronic equivalent for Schedule II drugs
B. State health certificate
C. Manufacturer's rebate form
D. Patient authorization form

Q155. Which act requires that medications be both pure and accurately labeled before distribution?

A. Pure Food and Drug Act of 1906
B. Food, Drug, and Cosmetic Act of 1938
C. Controlled Substances Act
D. Durham-Humphrey Amendment

Q156. What are the requirements for filing controlled substance records in a pharmacy?

A. File only by patient name
B. Combine all records alphabetically
C. Separate Schedule II from III–V and non-controlled records
D. Keep records with financial receipts

Q157. A patient requests a non-child-resistant cap for their medication. What must the pharmacy do?

A. Obtain a signed waiver from the patient
B. Refuse the request under any condition
C. Apply for FDA authorization
D. Remove the medication from the package

Q158. What does the term "readily retrievable" mean regarding controlled substance records?

A. Records are stored off-site indefinitely
B. Records can be produced within a short time for inspection
C. Records are only in paper format
D. Records can be destroyed after one year

Q159. When must a pharmacist report a significant loss of controlled substances to the DEA?

A. Within one business day of discovery
B. Within 30 days of audit
C. Only during annual inventory
D. Immediately after patient complaint

Q160. Which federal law established the Drug Enforcement Administration (DEA)?

A. Controlled Substances Act of 1970
B. Food, Drug, and Cosmetic Act of 1938
C. Harrison Narcotic Act
D. Poison Prevention Packaging Act

Q161. A pharmacist dispenses methadone for opioid addiction treatment. What requirement must be met?

A. No federal restrictions apply
B. Dispensed only by hospital emergency rooms
C. Dispensed through a DEA-registered opioid treatment program
D. Prescribed only for pain management

Q162. What type of notice must pharmacies provide when HIPAA policies change?

A. Revised Notice of Privacy Practices (NPP)
B. New patient consent forms only
C. DEA registration update
D. Insurance billing update

Q163. A pharmacist suspects elder abuse during patient counseling. What action is required?
A. Report suspicion to adult protective services immediately
B. Wait for patient consent before reporting
C. Only inform the patient's physician
D. Document but take no action
Q164. Under which conditions may an emergency refill of a Schedule III–V drug be provided without prescriber authorization?
A. When insurance allows extra fills
B. When a patient demands early refill
C. When the prescription has expired
D. When interruption may harm the patient and reasonable effort to contact the prescriber has been made
Q165. What is the primary objective of state pharmacy boards regarding controlled substance regulation?
A. Enforce state-specific pharmacy laws and discipline licensees
B. Approve drug advertisements
C. Manage federal labeling standards
D. Supervise DEA operations
Q166. Which federal agency oversees billing and reimbursement compliance for Medicare and Medicaid services within pharmacies?
A. OSHA
B. CMS
C. DEA
D. FDA
Q167. Under HIPAA regulations, which action is considered a breach of patient confidentiality?
A. Discussing medication therapy with the patient's authorized caregiver
B. Sharing PHI without consent to a non-clinical coworker
C. Reporting adverse drug events to the FDA
D. Counseling patients in a private area
Q168. The Omnibus Budget Reconciliation Act (OBRA) of 1990 primarily ensures what aspect of pharmacy practice?
A. Controlled substance tracking
B. Patient counseling and drug utilization review
C. Labeling and packaging compliance
D. Advertising restrictions for OTC drugs
Q169. Which organization provides national infection prevention guidelines relevant to pharmacy sterile compounding areas?
A. CDC
B. DEA
C. CMS
D. FDA
Q170. What is the main goal of the Controlled Substances Act (CSA)?
A. Encourage over-the-counter sales of narcotics
B. Regulate pharmacy insurance audits
C. Prevent misuse and diversion of controlled drugs
D. Establish packaging requirements
Q171. Under CMS policies, what defines a "high-cost outlier" claim in Medicare billing?
A. Any prescription exceeding a $500 cost threshold
B. A claim where cost surpasses standard reimbursement plus fixed loss amount

C. Prescriptions involving controlled substances
D. Claims denied for noncompliance

Q172. What law prohibits discrimination in healthcare settings receiving federal assistance?
A. Civil Rights Act of 1964
B. Controlled Substances Act
C. Food, Drug, and Cosmetic Act
D. HIPAA

Q173. Which entity oversees immunization program funding and distribution for community pharmacies?
A. CMS
B. CDC
C. DEA
D. OSHA

Q174. Which regulation outlines proper disposal of hazardous pharmaceutical waste?
A. Resource Conservation and Recovery Act (RCRA)
B. Controlled Substances Act
C. HIPAA
D. Food, Drug, and Cosmetic Act

Q175. A pharmacy technician notices a coworker removing medication samples without authorization. What should they do first?
A. Ignore the incident
B. Report to the supervising pharmacist
C. Confront the coworker directly
D. Call law enforcement immediately

Q176. Which law regulates the labeling of prescription and OTC drugs to ensure consumer safety?
A. Food, Drug, and Cosmetic Act
B. OBRA 1990
C. Poison Prevention Packaging Act
D. HIPAA

Q177. Under OSHA, what must pharmacies provide to employees exposed to hazardous materials?
A. Free immunizations
B. Legal immunity
C. Paid leave
D. Material Safety Data Sheets (MSDS) and training

Q178. What is the purpose of the Poison Prevention Packaging Act (PPPA)?
A. To control over-theprescribing of antibiotics
B. To reduce accidental poisonings via child-resistant packaging
C. To manage controlled substance scheduling
D. To enforce manufacturer recalls

Q179. Under the Affordable Care Act (ACA), pharmacies participating in federal programs must:
A. Offer all drugs at discounted prices
B. Maintain patient record confidentiality and access equity
C. Report only controlled drug sales
D. Limit counseling to insured patients

Q180. A technician is asked to release patient data for marketing purposes. Which law prohibits this without written authorization?
A. HIPAA
B. OBRA

C. CMS
D. RCRA

Q181. Which class of drugs is primarily used to lower blood pressure by relaxing blood vessels?
A. Beta-blockers
B. ACE inhibitors
C. Antacids
D. Diuretics

Q182. What is the mechanism of action of beta-blockers like metoprolol?
A. Stimulate adrenergic receptors to increase heart rate
B. Block beta-adrenergic receptors to slow heart rate and reduce blood pressure
C. Increase renin production to constrict blood vessels
D. Promote sodium reabsorption in kidneys

Q183. Which of the following medications is classified as a loop diuretic?
A. Hydrochlorothiazide
B. Spironolactone
C. Furosemide
D. Lisinopril

Q184. Which antibiotic class inhibits bacterial cell wall synthesis?
A. Macrolides
B. Penicillins
C. Tetracyclines
D. Fluoroquinolones

Q185. Which drug is considered a proton pump inhibitor (PPI)?
A. Ranitidine
B. Omeprazole
C. Famotidine
D. Sucralfate

Q186. What is the therapeutic purpose of statin medications like atorvastatin?
A. Lower blood glucose levels
B. Reduce cholesterol synthesis in the liver
C. Increase blood clotting
D. Relieve inflammation

Q187. Which neurotransmitter's reuptake is inhibited by SSRIs such as sertraline?
A. Dopamine
B. Acetylcholine
C. Serotonin
D. Norepinephrine

Q188. What is the primary side effect concern for patients taking loop diuretics like furosemide?
A. Hyperkalemia
B. Hypokalemia
C. Hyponatremia
D. Constipation

Q189. Which insulin type is rapid-acting and typically administered just before meals?
A. NPH
B. Regular insulin
C. Insulin lispro
D. Insulin glargine

Q190. What is the mechanism of action of calcium channel blockers like amlodipine?

A. Increase heart contractility
B. Block calcium influx in vascular smooth muscle
C. Stimulate adrenergic receptors
D. Inhibit angiotensin-converting enzyme

Q191. Which anticoagulant's effect is routinely monitored using the INR (International Normalized Ratio)?
A. Warfarin
B. Heparin
C. Dabigatran
D. Apixaban

Q192. Which antibiotic interaction can potentiate warfarin's anticoagulant effect, increasing bleeding risk?
A. Amoxicillin
B. Ciprofloxacin
C. Doxycycline
D. Azithromycin

Q193. Which class of inhaled medication is first-line for quick relief of acute bronchospasm?
A. Inhaled corticosteroids
B. Short-acting beta-agonists (SABA)
C. Long-acting muscarinic antagonists
D. Leukotriene modifiers

Q194. Which opioid is considered a strong opioid commonly used for severe pain management in acute settings?
A. Codeine
B. Morphine
C. Tramadol
D. Loperamide

Q195. What is a common gastrointestinal adverse effect associated with NSAIDs such as ibuprofen?
A. Constipation
B. Increased appetite
C. Peptic ulceration and GI bleeding
D. Hypoglycemia

Q196. Which vaccine type is generally contraindicated in severely immunocompromised patients?
A. Inactivated influenza vaccine
B. Tetanus toxoid vaccine
C. Live attenuated vaccines (e.g., MMR, varicella)
D. Hepatitis B vaccine

Q197. Which antiplatelet agent irreversibly inhibits the P2Y12 receptor on platelets and reduces thrombotic risk?
A. Aspirin
B. Clopidogrel
C. Warfarin
D. Heparin

Q198. Levodopa is co-administered with carbidopa primarily to:
A. Enhance peripheral conversion to dopamine
B. Prevent peripheral metabolism of levodopa, increasing central availability
C. Inhibit central dopamine receptors
D. Reduce serotonin levels

Q199. Which benzodiazepine is commonly used for acute seizure control in emergency settings?
A. Diazepam
B. Midazolam
C. Alprazolam
D. Lorazepam

Q200. Isotretinoin therapy requires strict pregnancy prevention due to which primary safety concern?
A. Hepatotoxicity
B. Teratogenicity causing severe fetal malformations
C. Gastrointestinal upset
D. Photosensitivity

Answer keys and Explanations (101-200)

Q101. Answer: A

Explanation: A valid controlled substance prescription must include the prescriber's signature (or electronic signature) and DEA number to confirm legal authority to prescribe controlled substances. The DEA number links the clinician to registration databases and helps prevent unauthorized prescribing. Pharmacy initials, insurance copies, or manufacturer lot numbers do not establish prescriber authority. Accurate prescriber identification assists in auditing, transfers, and detecting potential diversion.

Q102. Answer: A

Explanation: PHI encompasses individually identifiable health information tied to a person, including name, diagnosis, medical history, and contact details. Patient name linked with diagnosis constitutes PHI and is protected under HIPAA privacy rules. Pharmacy inventory, NDC codes, and expiration dates are not PHI unless linked to specific patient identifiers. Technicians must safeguard PHI, disclose only for permitted purposes, and follow employer policies to maintain confidentiality.

Q103. Answer: C

Explanation: OBRA 1990 mandates that pharmacists offer counseling to Medicaid patients to promote proper medication use and reduce adverse outcomes. It requires prospective drug utilization review and patient interaction to address drug therapy concerns, adherence, and safety. This federal requirement focuses specifically on Medicaid beneficiaries, but many pharmacies extend counseling services to all patients. Other listed acts target packaging, controlled substances, and drug safety/regulation rather than counseling obligations.

Q104. Answer: A

Explanation: The DSCSA establishes requirements for product tracing, verification, and detection of illegitimate prescription drugs in the supply chain, enabling rapid identification and removal of suspect products. It requires transaction records between manufacturers, wholesale distributors, and dispensers to enhance supply chain security. This law targets serialization, tracing, and reporting rather than packaging mandates, OTC sales restrictions, or formulary creation, thereby reducing counterfeit and diverted medications.

Q105. Answer: A

Explanation: Schedule II controlled substances require strict inventory control, typically through a perpetual inventory system that records each receipt and dispensation to maintain an accurate, up-to-date count. Federal regulations and DEA expectations call for precise tracking to prevent diversion, support investigations, and comply with recordkeeping standards. Annual counts alone are insufficient for Schedule II drugs, and they must be stored securely separate from OTC stock with access controls.

Q106. Answer: B

Explanation: Federal regulations permit the transfer of Schedule III–V prescriptions between pharmacies only once for refill purposes, to ensure proper oversight and prevent multiple duplicative transfers. This single-transfer rule helps maintain chain-of-custody records and prevents abuse. Transfers do not require DEA Form 222 (used for Schedule II ordering), and transfers are allowed but limited, unlike Schedule II prescriptions, which have stricter transfer rules.

Q107. Answer: A

Explanation: USP <800> provides standards for handling hazardous drugs to minimize exposure risks to healthcare personnel, patients, and the environment, detailing engineering controls, PPE, and disposal procedures. It complements other safety regulations and is widely adopted by pharmacies and health systems. The CSA regulates controlled substances, HIPAA covers privacy, and the PPPA addresses child-resistant packaging; none specifically govern hazardous drug handling protocols.

Q108. Answer: A

Explanation: Pharmacies must refuse to fill forged prescriptions, secure the document, notify the supervising pharmacist immediately, and report suspected fraud or diversion to law enforcement and the

DEA as appropriate. Filling forged prescriptions or altering prescriber information is illegal and may implicate pharmacy staff. Proper chain of custody and reporting protect patients and deter criminal activity while complying with federal and state regulations.

Q109. Answer: D

Explanation: Discrepancies that suggest diversion require immediate action: initiate an internal investigation to reconcile records, notify the pharmacist-in-charge, secure implicated inventory, and if theft or significant loss is suspected, report to the DEA via Form 106. Proper documentation, timely reporting, and corrective measures preserve public safety and regulatory compliance. Ignoring, destroying without records, or returning stock without documentation would violate regulations and impede investigations.

Q110. Answer: A

Explanation: The National Provider Identifier (NPI) is the standard unique identifier for healthcare providers used in electronic transactions, including billing Medicare Part D prescriptions. NPIs streamline claims processing and help protect patient data during electronic exchanges. Social Security numbers and employee badges are inappropriate for billing, while state license numbers may be used for professional credentialing but are not the standardized billing identifier required for Medicare claims.

Q111. Answer: A

Explanation: The CSA and associated DEA regulations require pharmacies to document receipt, return, transfer, and destruction of controlled substances, maintaining records for inspection and accountability. Proper documentation ensures traceability and compliance with diversion prevention measures. HIPAA governs privacy, the PPPA addresses packaging, and FLSA concerns labor standards; none mandate controlled substance return/destruction recordkeeping as the CSA and DEA do.

Q112. Answer: B

Explanation: A compliant prescription label must include patient name, drug name and strength, directions for use, prescriber's name, pharmacy name/address, and other required information to ensure safe use and regulatory compliance. These elements allow identification, proper administration, and enable pharmacists and patients to verify accuracy. Minimal labeling like only drug name or manufacturer details is insufficient and could jeopardize patient safety and violate state or federal labeling requirements.

Q113. Answer: A

Explanation: HIPAA permits disclosure of PHI without explicit patient authorization for purposes of treatment, payment, and healthcare operations, enabling necessary care coordination, billing, and quality improvement. Disclosures for marketing, public posting, or sharing SSNs with employers require authorization or are prohibited. Technicians must follow minimum-necessary standards and organizational policies when handling PHI to protect privacy and maintain compliance.

Q114. Answer: A

Explanation: The FDA MedWatch Form 3500 is used to report serious adverse events, product quality problems, medication errors, and other safety concerns associated with medical products. Reporting supports post-marketing surveillance and can prompt safety communications or recalls. DEA Form 222 handles Schedule II transactions, CMS-1500 supports billing, and OSHA Form 300 logs workplace injuries; none serve FDA adverse event reporting purposes.

Q115. Answer: C

Explanation: The PPPA requires child-resistant packaging for many prescription and nonprescription drugs to reduce pediatric poisoning incidents. It specifies performance standards for containers and allows certain exemptions (e.g., patient-requested non-child-resistant packaging). HIPAA addresses privacy, DSCSA addresses supply chain security, and OSHA focuses on workplace hazard communication rather than consumer packaging safety.

Q116. Answer: B

Explanation: The CSA was enacted to regulate and control the manufacture, distribution, and dispensing of controlled substances that have potential for abuse or dependency. It establishes schedules based on abuse potential and medical use, assigns DEA authority, and requires recordkeeping for compliance. The act does not govern dietary supplements or general food safety, which are regulated by other agencies such as the FDA or USDA.

Q117. Answer: A

Explanation: DEA Form 41 documents the destruction of controlled substances that are expired, damaged, or otherwise unsaleable. It requires details on drug name, strength, quantity, and method of destruction, ensuring accountability and proper waste disposal. Form 222 is for ordering, Form 106 reports theft or loss, and Form 224 is for registration, distinguishing each form's unique regulatory purpose in DEA compliance.

Q118. Answer: B

Explanation: DEA registration for pharmacies must be renewed every three years using DEA Form 224a. This ensures continuous authorization to handle controlled substances and maintains current records for auditing and inspection. The renewal process verifies ongoing compliance with regulations. Annual or five-year renewals are incorrect, and failing to renew on time may result in suspension of controlled substance handling privileges.

Q119. Answer: A

Explanation: Expired Schedule II medications must be transferred to a DEA-authorized reverse distributor for proper destruction and documentation using DEA Form 41. This ensures secure disposal, traceability, and environmental safety. Pharmacies cannot dispose of these drugs independently or return them to patients. Improper disposal, such as flushing or discarding, violates DEA and environmental regulations designed to prevent diversion and contamination.

Q120. Answer: A

Explanation: The Combat Methamphetamine Epidemic Act of 2005 limits retail sales of pseudoephedrine, ephedrine, and phenylpropanolamine, requiring identification, logbooks, and purchase limits. These substances are precursors in methamphetamine production, so strict regulation helps reduce illegal synthesis. The law doesn't apply to common analgesics or antihistamines like ibuprofen or loratadine. Technicians must ensure compliance with recordkeeping and daily quantity restrictions.

Q121. Answer: D

Explanation: Federal law limits retail sales of pseudoephedrine to 3.6 grams per person per day and 9 grams per 30 days. This restriction is part of the Combat Methamphetamine Epidemic Act to prevent bulk diversion for illegal drug manufacturing. Pharmacies must verify identification and maintain electronic or written logs. Exceeding limits or failing to record purchases violates federal compliance requirements.

Q122. Answer: B

Explanation: In emergency situations, Schedule II prescriptions may be phoned in, but the prescriber must provide a signed written or electronic prescription within seven days. The pharmacist must document the emergency, verify prescriber identity, and attach the written copy upon receipt. Failure to obtain the written order within the timeframe must be reported to the DEA. Longer delays violate federal dispensing regulations.

Q123. Answer: A

Explanation: Schedule II controlled substances must be stored in a securely locked, substantially constructed cabinet or safe to prevent unauthorized access. Leaving them in an unlocked cabinet violates DEA regulations and increases diversion risk. Schedule III–V drugs may be stored securely with general stock, provided monitoring systems exist. Maintaining daily checks supports compliance and loss prevention but doesn't replace secure physical storage.

Q124. Answer: A

Explanation: The 1962 Kefauver-Harris Amendment to the FD&C Act requires manufacturers to prove both safety and efficacy before a new drug can be marketed. It was passed following the thalidomide tragedy, reinforcing pre-market clinical testing and post-market surveillance. The Durham-Humphrey Amendment defines prescription vs. OTC drugs, while the CSA and DSCSA address controlled substances and supply chain security, not efficacy requirements.

Q125. Answer: C

Explanation: The 1951 Durham-Humphrey Amendment created the legal distinction between prescription (legend) drugs and over-the-counter (OTC) drugs. It authorized verbal prescriptions, refills, and required labeling stating "Caution: Federal law prohibits dispensing without prescription." This amendment clarified pharmacist and prescriber roles. It does not define controlled substance scheduling or labeling differences between brand and generic medications, which are covered by other laws.

Q126. Answer: A

Explanation: The FDA assigns National Drug Codes (NDCs), unique 10-digit identifiers used to track drug products. The first segment identifies the manufacturer, the second denotes product specifics, and the third describes packaging. This coding system supports recalls, reimbursement, and inventory management. DEA controls scheduling and registration, while CMS manages healthcare programs, and USP establishes quality and compounding standards, not product identification codes.

Q127. Answer: B

Explanation: Federal law requires pharmacies to conduct a complete controlled substance inventory at least every two years. This biennial inventory includes physical counts of Schedule II drugs and estimated counts for Schedules III–V (unless open containers exceed 1,000 units). The record must be dated, signed, and readily retrievable. Performing inventories more frequently is permissible but not mandated by federal regulation.

Q128. Answer: A

Explanation: DEA Form 106 must be completed when theft or significant loss of controlled substances occurs. It details the circumstances, quantities, and types of drugs involved. Prompt submission to the DEA and local authorities helps investigate and prevent diversion. Form 41 covers destruction, Form 222 handles Schedule II transfers, and Form 224 registers facilities, making Form 106 the designated loss-reporting document.

Q129. Answer: A

Explanation: The MedWatch program enables healthcare professionals and consumers to voluntarily report serious adverse events, product defects, and medication errors to the FDA. These reports support post-marketing surveillance and can trigger safety alerts, labeling updates, or recalls. MedWatch doesn't regulate controlled substances or inspections; it focuses solely on identifying safety trends and protecting public health through data collection and review.

Q130. Answer: A

Explanation: Phase I clinical trials involve small groups of healthy volunteers to evaluate drug safety, pharmacokinetics, and appropriate dosage ranges. This stage identifies adverse effects before proceeding to efficacy testing. Phase II assesses effectiveness in patients, Phase III confirms results in larger populations, and Phase IV monitors long-term effects post-approval. Early safety determination prevents broader exposure to potentially harmful compounds.

Q131. Answer: D

Explanation: DEA Form 222 records for Schedule II controlled substance transactions must be retained and readily available for inspection for at least two years from the date of final entry. These forms verify legitimate distribution and allow the DEA to audit compliance. Failing to maintain accessible documentation can result in penalties or loss of registration. Expiration or fulfillment does not negate recordkeeping obligations.

Q132. Answer: A

Explanation: To dispense controlled substances electronically, a pharmacy must maintain a valid DEA registration and use a DEA-approved, certified electronic prescription system. These systems authenticate prescribers, prevent forgery, and ensure compliance with federal e-prescribing regulations. HIPAA authorization, retail permits, or verbal approvals alone do not satisfy security or legal standards for transmitting controlled substance prescriptions electronically.

Q133. Answer: A

Explanation: The 1938 Food, Drug, and Cosmetic Act required drug manufacturers to prove product safety before marketing, following the sulfanilamide tragedy. It expanded FDA authority and established pre-market approval for new drugs. The 1906 Pure Food and Drug Act addressed labeling and adulteration, while the Kefauver-Harris Amendment later added efficacy requirements, and the CSA dealt with controlled substances regulation, not pre-market safety.

Q134. Answer: C

Explanation: The Prescription Drug Marketing Act (PDMA) of 1987 prohibits false or misleading advertising, restricts drug sample distribution, and prevents counterfeit and diverted prescription drugs from entering the supply chain. It safeguards drug integrity and protects consumers. While the FDA enforces labeling rules under the FD&C Act, and the FTC regulates OTC ads, the PDMA focuses on truthful prescription drug marketing and distribution integrity.

Q135. Answer: A

Explanation: The Child Abuse Prevention and Treatment Act (CAPTA) requires healthcare professionals, including pharmacy staff, to report suspected child abuse or neglect to appropriate authorities. This ensures timely intervention and protection of minors. HIPAA permits such disclosures without patient consent for safety reasons. CSA governs controlled substances, and OSHA regulates workplace safety, making CAPTA the key law for mandatory child protection reporting.

Q136. Answer: B

Explanation: Schedule V substances, such as certain cough syrups containing limited codeine, have the lowest abuse potential among controlled substances and may be available without prescription under specific state laws. They do not require DEA Form 222 and may be refilled per standard prescription regulations. These medications retain medical use for humans, distinguishing them from restricted or higher-schedule substances requiring stricter controls.

Q137. Answer: A

Explanation: The pharmacist holds ultimate responsibility for verifying the validity of DEA registration numbers on controlled substance prescriptions. Verification ensures prescriber legitimacy and prevents fraudulent dispensing. While technicians may assist in preliminary checks, only the pharmacist can authorize dispensing. Patients and office assistants lack legal authority or access to validate DEA credentials, making pharmacist oversight essential for compliance and security.

Q138. Answer: C

Explanation: Alprazolam (Xanax) is a Schedule IV controlled substance under the DEA, indicating a lower abuse potential compared to Schedules I–III but higher than Schedule V. It is commonly prescribed for anxiety and panic disorders. Schedule IV drugs may be refilled up to five times in six months. Schedule II substances have stricter refill and prescribing limitations due to higher abuse risk.

Q139. Answer: A

Explanation: DEA Form 224 is required for pharmacies, hospitals, and practitioners seeking initial registration to handle controlled substances. This form establishes authorization under the Controlled Substances Act and must be renewed every three years. Form 222 is used for ordering Schedule II drugs, Form 106 reports theft, and Form 41 documents destruction, distinguishing Form 224 as the registration application document.

Q140. Answer: A

Explanation: The Consumer Product Safety Commission (CPSC) enforces the Poison Prevention Packaging Act, which mandates child-resistant packaging for prescription and over-the-counter medications to prevent accidental poisoning. The CPSC sets performance standards and handles enforcement actions.

The FDA regulates drug safety, the DEA oversees controlled substances, and the CDC focuses on public health surveillance rather than packaging compliance.

Q141. Answer: D

Explanation: The Controlled Substances Ordering System (CSOS) allows registrants to electronically order Schedule II–V controlled substances securely, replacing paper DEA Form 222 for efficiency. CSOS uses digital certificates for authentication and recordkeeping, reducing errors and turnaround time. It does not report thefts or medication errors. CSOS ensures compliance, accuracy, and traceability across the controlled substance supply chain.

Q142. Answer: A

Explanation: DEA Form 222 must accompany any transfer of Schedule II controlled substances between DEA registrants, including pharmacies, distributors, and reverse distributors. It verifies the legitimacy of the transaction and ensures regulatory traceability. DEA Form 41 covers destruction, Form 106 covers theft, and Form 224 registers entities. Proper completion and filing of Form 222 prevent diversion and maintain compliance with DEA regulations.

Q143. Answer: B

Explanation: A pharmacy must renew its DEA registration every three years using Form 224a to continue dispensing controlled substances. This renewal ensures ongoing compliance with federal requirements and maintains authorization for handling scheduled drugs. Renewal reminders are issued by the DEA before expiration. Failure to renew results in suspension of controlled substance privileges until registration is revalidated.

Q144. Answer: A

Explanation: The Durham-Humphrey Amendment of 1951 defined the distinction between prescription and over-the-counter medications, requiring "Caution: Federal law prohibits dispensing without prescription" labeling on legend drugs. It also permitted verbal prescriptions and refills. The other acts govern efficacy, marketing, and child-resistant packaging, making the Durham-Humphrey Amendment foundational to prescription labeling laws and pharmacist dispensing practices.

Q145. Answer: A

Explanation: Controlled substance prescription labels must contain essential identifying information including patient name, pharmacy details, prescription number, date, prescriber, drug name, strength, and directions for use. These details support safe administration, verification, and regulatory compliance. DEA numbers are required for prescriber identification but not printed on labels. Insurance or pricing information is optional and not mandated by federal regulations.

Q146. Answer: C

Explanation: The DEA enforces the Controlled Substances Act, regulating manufacture, distribution, and dispensing of controlled substances to prevent abuse and diversion. It registers entities, conducts inspections, and monitors prescription use. The FDA ensures drug safety and labeling accuracy, CMS manages reimbursement programs, and the CPSC handles product safety; none have direct enforcement authority over the CSA's controlled substance provisions.

Q147. Answer: A

Explanation: DEA regulations allow prescribers to issue multiple Schedule II prescriptions on the same day totaling up to a 90-day supply, provided each prescription has a legitimate medical purpose and a specified "do not fill before" date. This practice prevents patient interruptions while maintaining regulatory compliance. Unauthorized multiple prescriptions or backdating would violate DEA dispensing laws and invite disciplinary action.

Q148. Answer: A

Explanation: The FDA's CDER ensures that prescription and over-the-counter drugs marketed in the United States are safe, effective, and properly labeled. It reviews clinical trial data, approves new drugs, and monitors post-marketing safety. CDER does not regulate medical devices, food labeling, or workplace safety. Its scientific evaluations form the basis for public drug safety assurance.

Q149. Answer: B

Explanation: Pharmacies must ensure that the DEA registration certificate posted on premises accurately lists the registrant's name, address, and registration expiration date. This verifies authorization to handle controlled substances at that location. Inaccurate or expired certificates can result in penalties. Continuing education, drug expiration, and employee logs are unrelated to DEA registration requirements for pharmacy operation compliance.

Q150. Answer: A

Explanation: The Controlled Substances Act mandates that all records related to controlled substances—including inventories, prescriptions, and transfers—be maintained and readily retrievable for DEA inspection. This ensures transparency and accountability in handling controlled drugs. HIPAA governs privacy, while PPPA and PDMA address packaging and marketing. Only the CSA enforces accessible, detailed recordkeeping requirements for controlled substances.

Q151. Answer: A

Explanation: DEA numbers beginning with "X" identify prescribers authorized under the Drug Addiction Treatment Act (DATA 2000) to prescribe buprenorphine and similar medications for opioid dependency treatment. This helps distinguish qualified practitioners in medication-assisted therapy programs. The "X" does not relate to DEA employment or veterinary limitation, and Schedule I substances remain prohibited for prescription use.

Q152. Answer: D

Explanation: Hospitals must secure controlled substances in locked, substantially constructed cabinets accessible only to authorized personnel. Security policies and periodic audits prevent diversion. Open or unlocked storage violates DEA and hospital compliance protocols. Integrating electronic access systems with physical controls ensures accountability, aligns with DEA standards, and reduces risk of theft or unauthorized use within institutional pharmacies.

Q153. Answer: A

Explanation: Each controlled substance dispensing transaction must include documentation of the date, quantity dispensed, prescription number, and initials or signature of the dispensing pharmacist. Immediate documentation ensures accurate tracking and compliance with DEA audit requirements. Insurance details and external supplier information are not mandated at dispensing, as the focus remains on accountability for controlled drug quantities and professional oversight.

Q154. Answer: A

Explanation: When transferring Schedule II controlled substances to a reverse distributor, the sending pharmacy must include DEA Form 222 or an approved electronic equivalent. This verifies legal custody transfer and facilitates destruction documentation. Schedules III–V require invoices instead. State health certificates, rebates, or patient authorization forms are irrelevant to DEA transfer requirements and do not meet controlled substance chain-of-custody standards.

Q155. Answer: A

Explanation: The Pure Food and Drug Act of 1906 was the first major consumer protection law, prohibiting interstate commerce of adulterated or misbranded drugs and foods. It established the foundation for modern FDA oversight, ensuring products met purity and labeling standards. Later laws expanded these protections to include safety, efficacy, and classification criteria for drugs, strengthening pharmaceutical regulation.

Q156. Answer: C

Explanation: Federal law requires pharmacies to maintain separate files for Schedule II records, while Schedules III–V may be filed together or separately from non-controlled prescriptions if clearly marked. This organization allows DEA inspectors to identify controlled substance records quickly. Mixing all prescriptions alphabetically or combining with unrelated records violates federal retrieval standards and complicates audits and regulatory inspections.

Q157. Answer: A

Explanation: Under the Poison Prevention Packaging Act, patients may request non-child-resistant packaging if they sign a waiver acknowledging the risk. This protects the pharmacy legally while respecting patient preference. Pharmacists should retain the waiver in records for verification. The request cannot be granted without documentation, as compliance ensures safety standards and prevents misuse or accidental ingestion by children.

Q158. Answer: B

Explanation: "Readily retrievable" means controlled substance records can be accessed quickly and efficiently for DEA inspection, whether maintained electronically or on paper. They must be organized, indexed, and available without delay during audits. Off-site storage or premature destruction violates compliance standards. The definition emphasizes accessibility and traceability to ensure accountability for all controlled substance transactions.

Q159. Answer: A

Explanation: DEA regulations require pharmacies to report any significant theft or loss of controlled substances to the DEA within one business day of discovery using Form 106. Prompt reporting enables investigation and mitigates diversion. Waiting until audits or patient complaints would delay corrective action and violate regulatory timelines, risking penalties for non-compliance under federal law.

Q160. Answer: A

Explanation: The Controlled Substances Act of 1970 established the Drug Enforcement Administration (DEA) to consolidate federal drug enforcement efforts and regulate controlled substances. It replaced earlier fragmented systems, setting national standards for scheduling, registration, and enforcement. The Harrison Act addressed narcotics taxation, and the FD&C Act focused on drug safety, but only the CSA created the DEA's unified authority.

Q161. Answer: C

Explanation: Methadone used for opioid addiction must be dispensed only through DEA-registered opioid treatment programs (OTPs) certified by SAMHSA. This ensures safe administration, monitoring, and compliance with federal law. Methadone for pain management follows standard prescribing rules, but addiction treatment is tightly regulated to prevent misuse. Unauthorized dispensing violates DEA and federal addiction treatment regulations.

Q162. Answer: A

Explanation: When HIPAA privacy policies change, pharmacies must provide patients with a revised Notice of Privacy Practices (NPP) detailing updated rights, uses, and disclosures of PHI. The notice must be available upon request and displayed prominently. DEA registration and insurance procedures are unrelated. The NPP ensures patients remain informed about how their health information is managed and protected.

Q163. Answer: A

Explanation: Pharmacists are mandatory reporters of elder abuse in most jurisdictions. Upon reasonable suspicion, they must immediately notify adult protective services or appropriate authorities. Waiting for patient consent or reporting only to a physician delays protection and violates state reporting laws. Documentation is essential, but prompt reporting ensures the safety and well-being of vulnerable adults.

Q164. Answer: D

Explanation: An emergency refill for Schedule III–V drugs may be provided if interrupting therapy could endanger the patient's health and the pharmacist has attempted but failed to contact the prescriber. Documentation must justify the decision, and only a limited supply should be dispensed. Filling expired prescriptions or providing refills on demand without clinical justification breaches legal and ethical pharmacy practice standards.

Q165. Answer: A

Explanation: State boards of pharmacy enforce state-level pharmacy laws, including those governing controlled substances, and ensure professional conduct among pharmacists and technicians. They conduct inspections, investigate violations, and impose disciplinary actions when needed. Federal labeling and DEA operations remain outside their jurisdiction, though boards often collaborate with the DEA to uphold both state and federal regulatory compliance.

Q166. Answer: B

Explanation: CMS regulates Medicare and Medicaid billing integrity, ensuring pharmacies maintain accurate claim submissions and prevent fraudulent activities. DEA and FDA primarily manage drug control and safety, while OSHA governs workplace safety. CMS focuses specifically on reimbursement accuracy and healthcare service compliance, making it central to pharmacy operations involving government insurance.

Q167. Answer: B

Explanation: Sharing PHI without authorization violates HIPAA privacy standards designed to protect personal medical information. Authorized communication and safety reporting to regulatory bodies are permissible, as they support patient care and safety. Only disclosure without consent or valid reason constitutes a privacy breach.

Q168. Answer: B

Explanation: OBRA '90 mandates pharmacists to provide patient counseling and conduct drug utilization reviews to prevent medication errors. It enhances patient safety and therapeutic effectiveness by promoting communication. Unlike DEA or FDA oversight, OBRA focuses on patient-centered pharmacy practice within Medicaid and broader patient care.

Q169. Answer: A

Explanation: The CDC publishes infection control guidelines, including practices applied to sterile compounding and immunization safety. DEA handles controlled substances, CMS manages reimbursement systems, and FDA regulates drug approval. Infection control remains within CDC's expertise, ensuring health safety standards.

Q170. Answer: C

Explanation: The CSA prevents abuse and diversion of controlled drugs by classifying substances into schedules and setting strict distribution controls. This ensures accountability from manufacturers to dispensers. Other agencies handle insurance and labeling, but the CSA's foundation is drug abuse prevention.

Q171. Answer: B

Explanation: A high-cost outlier claim exceeds the regular payment and the fixed-loss threshold, triggering additional reimbursement. CMS uses this mechanism to balance fair payments for unusually expensive cases, ensuring providers aren't financially penalized for legitimate, high-cost treatments.

Q172. Answer: A

Explanation: The Civil Rights Act prohibits discrimination based on race, color, or national origin in facilities receiving federal funding. In pharmacy contexts, this ensures equitable treatment and access for all patients. Other laws address drug safety or privacy but not civil equality.

Q173. Answer: B

Explanation: The CDC coordinates immunization programs, ensuring proper vaccine storage, distribution, and data tracking in community settings. CMS manages billing, DEA controls substances, and OSHA regulates workplace safety. The CDC's involvement ensures vaccine program consistency and disease prevention.

Q174. Answer: A

Explanation: The RCRA establishes protocols for safe hazardous waste disposal, ensuring environmental protection and public health. It applies to pharmacies handling expired or cytotoxic drugs. Unlike HIPAA or DEA rules, RCRA focuses solely on environmental and waste management compliance.

Q175. Answer: B

Explanation: Technicians should promptly report suspected diversion or theft to the supervising pharmacist. The pharmacist is legally obligated to investigate and report to the DEA or authorities if warranted. Direct confrontation may escalate risk, while ignoring breaches violates ethical and legal standards.

Q176. Answer: A

Explanation: The FD&C Act ensures that all marketed drugs are accurately labeled and safe for intended use, covering both prescription and OTC items. OBRA addresses counseling, while the Poison Prevention Act focuses on packaging safety rather than label accuracy.

Q177. Answer: D

Explanation: OSHA mandates that employers maintain MSDS documentation and provide safety training for hazardous material exposure. This ensures informed handling and workplace safety. Immunizations or leave policies may apply separately but are not core OSHA requirements.

Q178. Answer: B

Explanation: The PPPA requires child-resistant packaging to minimize accidental poisonings, especially among children. It mandates secure container designs for certain medications. It differs from DEA scheduling or recall enforcement, which fall under other laws.

Q179. Answer: B

Explanation: The ACA enforces equity in patient access and privacy, ensuring participating pharmacies maintain confidentiality while offering nondiscriminatory services. It strengthens patient protection through ethical and transparent healthcare delivery rather than pricing mandates.

Q180. Answer: A

Explanation: HIPAA explicitly forbids sharing PHI for marketing without explicit, documented patient consent. This ensures confidentiality and ethical data use. OBRA and RCRA govern patient care and waste disposal respectively, while CMS deals with reimbursement—not privacy.

Q181. Answer: B

Explanation: ACE inhibitors such as lisinopril prevent conversion of angiotensin I to angiotensin II, reducing vasoconstriction and aldosterone-mediated sodium retention. The resulting vasodilation decreases systemic vascular resistance and lowers blood pressure while reducing afterload on the heart. These agents are commonly used for hypertension and heart failure and have renal-protective effects in diabetic nephropathy; monitoring for cough and hyperkalemia is necessary.

Q182. Answer: B

Explanation: Beta-blockers antagonize beta-adrenergic receptors, primarily beta-1 in the heart, diminishing sympathetic-driven increases in heart rate and contractility. This lowers myocardial oxygen demand, controls arrhythmias, and reduces blood pressure. Metoprolol's cardioselectivity reduces bronchospastic risk compared with nonselective agents but still requires caution in reactive airway disease. Dose titration and monitoring for bradycardia and fatigue are standard practice.

Q183. Answer: C

Explanation: Furosemide is a potent loop diuretic that inhibits the Na-K-2Cl transporter in the thick ascending limb of the loop of Henle, markedly increasing sodium, chloride, and water excretion. It is useful for edema associated with heart failure, renal impairment, or hepatic disease. Because it can produce significant electrolyte disturbances, particularly hypokalemia and hypomagnesemia, patients require laboratory monitoring and sometimes supplemental potassium.

Q184. Answer: B

Explanation: Beta-lactam antibiotics such as penicillins block bacterial cell wall synthesis by binding penicillin-binding proteins and inhibiting peptidoglycan cross-linking, leading to cell lysis under osmotic stress. This mechanism is bactericidal and particularly effective against Gram-positive organisms. Resistance mechanisms include beta-lactamase production and altered PBPs. Clinicians select specific agents based on spectrum, allergy history, and local resistance patterns.

Q185. Answer: B

Explanation: Omeprazole is a proton pump inhibitor that irreversibly inhibits the H+/K+ ATPase enzyme in gastric parietal cells, reducing gastric acid secretion and raising gastric pH. PPIs are indicated for GERD, peptic ulcer disease, and H. pylori eradication protocols. Long-term use may be associated with risks such as nutrient malabsorption, increased fracture risk, and infections like C. difficile; periodic reassessment is recommended.

Q186. Answer: B

Explanation: Statins inhibit HMG-CoA reductase, the rate-limiting enzyme in hepatic cholesterol synthesis, decreasing intracellular cholesterol and upregulating LDL receptors to clear circulating LDL cholesterol. Reduced LDL levels lower atherosclerotic cardiovascular disease risk. Statins also have modest anti-inflammatory effects. Monitoring includes liver enzymes and assessment for myopathy; drug interactions (CYP3A4 inhibitors) can increase statin exposure and adverse effects.

Q187. Answer: C

Explanation: Selective serotonin reuptake inhibitors (SSRIs) block the serotonin transporter (SERT), reducing reabsorption of serotonin into presynaptic neurons and enhancing serotonergic neurotransmission. This modulation improves mood and anxiety symptoms over weeks of treatment. Common adverse effects include gastrointestinal upset, sexual dysfunction, and potential serotonin syndrome when combined with other serotonergic agents; clinicians monitor response and tolerability during initiation and dose changes.

Q188. Answer: B

Explanation: Loop diuretics increase urinary excretion of potassium, predisposing patients to hypokalemia, which may cause muscle weakness, cramps, and dangerous cardiac arrhythmias. Electrolyte monitoring and supplementation are often necessary, especially in patients on concurrent digoxin or with cardiac disease. Additionally, loop diuretics can cause volume depletion and renal function changes; careful dosing and lab surveillance help mitigate risks.

Q189. Answer: C

Explanation: Insulin lispro is a rapid-acting analogue with onset within 15 minutes, peak effect around one hour, and a short duration, matching prandial glucose excursions when administered immediately before meals. It reduces postprandial hyperglycemia and allows flexible mealtime dosing. Patients must coordinate carbohydrate intake and timing to avoid hypoglycemia; education on injection technique and hypoglycemia management is essential.

Q190. Answer: B

Explanation: Dihydropyridine calcium channel blockers such as amlodipine inhibit L-type calcium channels in vascular smooth muscle, causing vasodilation and reduced peripheral resistance, thereby lowering blood pressure. They primarily affect arterioles rather than cardiac conduction, making them effective antihypertensives with reflex tachycardia risk. Peripheral edema is a common adverse effect; dose adjustments and combination therapy may mitigate side effects.

Q191. Answer: A

Explanation: Warfarin, a vitamin K antagonist, requires routine monitoring via the INR to maintain therapeutic anticoagulation and balance bleeding risk. INR reflects the activity of vitamin K–dependent clotting factors and is affected by diet, drug interactions, and hepatic function. Frequent testing and dose adjustments are necessary to achieve target ranges for various indications; patient education on interactions and adherence is critical.

Q192. Answer: B

Explanation: Ciprofloxacin can inhibit cytochrome P450 enzymes involved in warfarin metabolism, leading to increased warfarin levels and elevated INR, thereby raising bleeding risk. Clinicians should monitor INR closely and consider warfarin dose adjustments when starting or stopping interacting antibiotics. While azithromycin and doxycycline have less pronounced effects, vigilance is needed for any antibiotic that may alter gut flora or hepatic metabolism affecting warfarin.

Q193. Answer: B

Explanation: Short-acting beta-agonists (SABAs) such as albuterol provide rapid bronchodilation by stimulating beta-2 receptors in bronchial smooth muscle, relieving acute bronchospasm within minutes. They are cornerstone rescue medications for asthma exacerbations and COPD symptom relief. Maintenance therapies (inhaled corticosteroids, long-acting bronchodilators) address inflammation and long-term control but do not replace SABAs for emergent relief.

Q194. Answer: B

Explanation: Morphine is a prototypical strong opioid agonist with high affinity for mu-opioid receptors, producing potent analgesia for severe acute and chronic pain. It carries significant risks including respiratory depression, sedation, and dependence, so dosing must be individualized with monitoring. Alternatives like codeine and tramadol are weaker and have different metabolic considerations; loperamide is an antidiarrheal with peripheral opioid activity.

Q195. Answer: C

Explanation: NSAIDs inhibit COX-1–mediated prostaglandin synthesis, reducing protective gastric mucosal defenses and increasing risk for peptic ulcers and gastrointestinal bleeding, particularly with prolonged use, high doses, or concomitant anticoagulant therapy. Clinicians should evaluate GI risk factors and consider gastroprotective strategies like PPIs, alternative analgesics, or lowest effective NSAID dosing to minimize complications.

Q196. Answer: C

Explanation: Live attenuated vaccines replicate to a limited degree and can pose infection risks in severely immunocompromised patients, including those on high-dose steroids or chemotherapy. Therefore, vaccines like MMR and varicella are typically contraindicated in this population. Inactivated, toxoid, and recombinant vaccines are preferred and safer; immunization decisions should consider individual immune status, timing, and specialist consultation.

Q197. Answer: B

Explanation: Clopidogrel irreversibly blocks the P2Y12 ADP receptor on platelets, preventing ADP-mediated platelet activation and aggregation. It reduces thrombotic risk in acute coronary syndromes and after stent placement. Because inhibition is irreversible, platelet function normalizes only as new platelets are produced; clinicians consider bleeding risk, drug interactions (e.g., proton pump inhibitors), and genetic variability affecting response.

Q198. Answer: B

Explanation: Carbidopa inhibits peripheral aromatic L-amino acid decarboxylase, preventing levodopa conversion to dopamine outside the CNS, thereby increasing levodopa's central availability and reducing peripheral adverse effects such as nausea and cardiovascular effects. This allows lower levodopa dosing to achieve therapeutic central dopamine levels for Parkinson's symptom control while minimizing systemic side effects and improving tolerability.

Q199. Answer: D

Explanation: Lorazepam is preferred for acute seizure termination due to its potency, relatively sustained anticonvulsant effect when given intravenously, and predictable pharmacokinetics. It is often the first-line agent in status epilepticus. Diazepam acts quickly but redistributes rapidly and may require repeat dosing, while midazolam is useful intramuscularly or intranasally in prehospital settings. Alprazolam is not indicated for emergencies.

Q200. Answer: B

Explanation: Isotretinoin carries a high teratogenic risk and can cause profound fetal malformations including craniofacial, cardiac, and central nervous system defects. Programs like iPLEDGE mandate negative pregnancy tests and reliable contraception before and during therapy to prevent exposure. While monitoring for hepatotoxicity and lipid abnormalities is required, preventing fetal exposure is the paramount safety concern due to irreversible outcomes.

```
```

Questions (201-300)

Q201. Which class of antidepressants includes medications such as amitriptyline and nortriptyline?
A. SSRIs
B. SNRIs
C. Tricyclic antidepressants (TCAs)
D. MAO inhibitors

Q202. What is the therapeutic use of the drug albuterol?
A. Antihistamine for allergies
B. Bronchodilator for asthma and COPD
C. Antitussive for cough
D. Corticosteroid for inflammation

Q203. What is the primary mechanism of metformin in treating type 2 diabetes?
A. Increases glucose uptake and decreases hepatic glucose production
B. Stimulates pancreatic insulin release
C. Slows carbohydrate absorption
D. Promotes insulin degradation

Q204. Which electrolyte imbalance is commonly caused by thiazide diuretics?
A. Hyperkalemia
B. Hypokalemia
C. Hypernatremia
D. Hypercalcemia

Q205. Which antibiotic class carries a black box warning for tendon rupture and neuropathy?
A. Macrolides
B. Fluoroquinolones
C. Aminoglycosides
D. Cephalosporins

Q206. What is the most common side effect of opioid analgesics such as oxycodone?
A. Diarrhea
B. Rash
C. Constipation
D. Tachycardia

Q207. Which antidiabetic medication stimulates insulin release from pancreatic beta cells?
A. Metformin
B. Glipizide
C. Pioglitazone
D. Acarbose

Q208. Which neurotransmitter imbalance is most associated with Parkinson's disease?
A. Dopamine deficiency
B. Acetylcholine excess
C. Serotonin deficiency
D. Norepinephrine excess

Q209. Which medication is commonly used as an anticoagulant for deep vein thrombosis prophylaxis in hospitalized patients?
A. Warfarin
B. Enoxaparin
C. Dabigatran
D. Clopidogrel

Q210. What is the mechanism of action of proton pump inhibitors such as pantoprazole?
A. Block H2 receptors on parietal cells
B. Neutralize stomach acid
C. Inhibit the gastric hydrogen-potassium ATPase enzyme
D. Stimulate mucus secretion
Q211. Which class of drugs is used as a first-line treatment for generalized anxiety disorder?
A. Benzodiazepines
B. SSRIs
C. Antipsychotics
D. MAO inhibitors
Q212. Which vaccine is recommended annually for most adults to prevent respiratory infection?
A. Pneumococcal
B. Influenza
C. Tdap
D. MMR
Q213. Which medication is classified as a selective estrogen receptor modulator (SERM) used for osteoporosis prevention?
A. Raloxifene
B. Alendronate
C. Calcitonin
D. Tamoxifen
Q214. Which medication is used to reverse opioid overdose?
A. Naloxone
B. Flumazenil
C. Naltrexone
D. Physostigmine
Q215. Which class of drugs is primarily used to manage heart failure by blocking angiotensin II receptors?
A. ACE inhibitors
B. Beta-blockers
C. Angiotensin II receptor blockers (ARBs)
D. Calcium channel blockers
Q216. What is the mechanism of action of benzodiazepines like lorazepam?
A. Enhance GABA activity at the GABA-A receptor
B. Inhibit NMDA receptors
C. Block dopamine reuptake
D. Stimulate serotonin release
Q217. Which class of antipsychotic drugs is associated with a lower risk of extrapyramidal side effects?
A. First-generation (typical) antipsychotics
B. Second-generation (atypical) antipsychotics
C. Tricyclic antidepressants
D. MAO inhibitors
Q218. Which common over-the-counter analgesic can cause liver toxicity when overdosed?
A. Ibuprofen
B. Acetaminophen
C. Aspirin
D. Naproxen
Q219. Which medication is used as a thyroid hormone replacement for hypothyroidism?

A. Levothyroxine
B. Methimazole
C. Liothyronine
D. Propylthiouracil

Q220. Which class of medications is primarily prescribed to treat hyperlipidemia when statins are contraindicated or insufficient?

A. Fibrates
B. Loop diuretics
C. Alpha-blockers
D. Beta-blockers

Q221. Which class of drugs reduces inflammation by inhibiting prostaglandin synthesis?

A. Corticosteroids
B. NSAIDs
C. Antihistamines
D. Beta-blockers

Q222. Which medication is commonly prescribed for gastroesophageal reflux disease (GERD)?

A. Metformin
B. Lisinopril
C. Loratadine
D. Omeprazole

Q223. What is the mechanism of action of angiotensin receptor blockers (ARBs)?

A. Inhibit angiotensin-converting enzyme
B. Block angiotensin II from binding to receptors
C. Promote sodium retention
D. Increase aldosterone secretion

Q224. Which antibiotic should be avoided in children due to risk of teeth discoloration?

A. Amoxicillin
B. Tetracycline
C. Cephalexin
D. Erythromycin

Q225. Which class of medications reduces LDL cholesterol by inhibiting intestinal cholesterol absorption?

A. Statins
B. Bile acid sequestrants
C. Ezetimibe
D. Fibrates

Q226. Which medication is used as an anticonvulsant and mood stabilizer in bipolar disorder?

A. Valproic acid
B. Fluoxetine
C. Phenytoin
D. Lithium

Q227. Which antihistamine causes minimal sedation and is preferred for daytime allergy relief?

A. Diphenhydramine
B. Cetirizine
C. Loratadine
D. Hydroxyzine

Q228. Which class of drugs is primarily used to treat fungal infections of the skin and nails?

A. Antivirals

B. Antifungals
C. Antibiotics
D. Anthelmintics

Q229. Which medication acts as an alpha-glucosidase inhibitor for diabetes management?
A. Acarbose
B. Pioglitazone
C. Glipizide
D. Metformin

Q230. Which medication is used to prevent gout attacks by lowering uric acid levels?
A. Allopurinol
B. Colchicine
C. Indomethacin
D. Naproxen

Q231. Which antipsychotic medication is known for causing agranulocytosis and requires regular blood monitoring?
A. Risperidone
B. Clozapine
C. Haloperidol
D. Quetiapine

Q232. Which drug class does amlodipine belong to?
A. Beta-blockers
B. ACE inhibitors
C. Calcium channel blockers
D. Alpha-blockers

Q233. What is the primary therapeutic use of nitroglycerin?
A. Treat hypertension
B. Relieve chest pain from angina
C. Prevent blood clots
D. Manage heart failure

Q234. Which antibiotic is commonly prescribed for urinary tract infections (UTIs)?
A. Ciprofloxacin
B. Vancomycin
C. Doxycycline
D.Wp Azithromycin

Q235. Which medication is used to manage chronic asthma by reducing airway inflammation?
A. Albuterol
B. Montelukast
C. Prednisone
D. Salmeterol

Q236. Which over-the-counter medication is a proton pump inhibitor used for frequent heartburn?
A. Ranitidine
B. Omeprazole
C. Sucralfate
D. Aluminum hydroxide

Q237. Which medication acts as a potassium-sparing diuretic used in combination therapy for hypertension?
A. Spironolactone
B. Furosemide

C. Hydrochlorothiazide
D. Bumetanide

Q238. Which insulin preparation provides long-acting basal coverage lasting up to 24 hours?

A. Insulin lispro
B. Insulin aspart
C. Insulin glargine
D. NPH insulin

Q239. Which medication is a skeletal muscle relaxant commonly used for acute musculoskeletal pain?

A. Cyclobenzaprine
B. Diazepam
C. Baclofen
D. Methocarbamol

Q240. Which medication is classified as an angiotensin-converting enzyme (ACE) inhibitor?

A. Losartan
B. Lisinopril
C. Diltiazem
D. Amlodipine

Q241. Which antibiotic is often used to treat Clostridioides difficile infections?

A. Vancomycin
B. Azithromycin
C. Ciprofloxacin
D. Doxycycline

Q242. Which class of drugs is used to treat chronic heart failure by increasing myocardial contractility?

A. Beta-blockers
B. Cardiac glycosides
C. Diuretics
D. ACE inhibitors

Q243. Which vaccine protects against human papillomavirus (HPV) infections associated with cervical cancer?

A. Hepatitis B vaccine
B. Tdap vaccine
C. Varicella vaccine
D. HPV vaccine

Q244. Which drug is an opioid antagonist used for maintenance therapy in opioid dependence?

A. Naloxone
B. Naltrexone
C. Methadone
D. Buprenorphine

Q245. Which medication is a selective beta-2 agonist used for long-term control of asthma?

A. Albuterol
B. Formoterol
C. Montelukast
D. Ipratropium

Q246. Which drug class is primarily indicated for the treatment of peptic ulcer disease caused by H. pylori infection?

A. Antacids alone
B. Antibiotics and proton pump inhibitors
C. Corticosteroids

D. H2 receptor blockers alone

Q247. Which antidiabetic medication belongs to the SGLT2 inhibitor class?

A. Glipizide
B. Canagliflozin
C. Metformin
D. Acarbose

Q248. Which medication is a benzodiazepine used as a preoperative sedative and for procedural anxiety?

A. Alprazolam
B. Lorazepam
C. Midazolam
D. Diazepam

Q249. Which drug is a dopamine antagonist used as an antiemetic for nausea and vomiting?

A. Ondansetron
B. Metoclopramide
C. Promethazine
D. Scopolamine

Q250. Which vitamin deficiency can lead to pernicious anemia?

A. Vitamin B12
B. Vitamin C
C. Vitamin D
D. Folic acid

Q251. Which class of drugs is used as the main therapy for chronic hypertension?

A. Antibiotics
B. Antihypertensives
C. Antivirals
D. Antiemetics

Q252. Which antipsychotic is associated with the lowest risk of metabolic side effects?

A. Olanzapine
B. Clozapine
C. Aripiprazole
D. Quetiapine

Q253. Which anticonvulsant medication requires regular monitoring of blood levels due to its narrow therapeutic index?

A. Phenytoin
B. Valproate
C. Carbamazepine
D. Lamotrigine

Q254. Which medication is an alpha-blocker used to improve urinary flow in benign prostatic hyperplasia (BPH)?

A. Tamsulosin
B. Finasteride
C. Doxazosin
D. Lisinopril

Q255. Which anti-inflammatory drug class works by inhibiting phospholipase A2 activity?

A. COX-2 inhibitors
B. NSAIDs
C. Antihistamines

D. Corticosteroids

Q256. Which drug is a mucolytic agent used to thin respiratory secretions in chronic lung disease?

A. Albuterol
B. Acetylcysteine
C. Montelukast
D. Diphenhydramine

Q257. Which medication is classified as a bisphosphonate used to treat osteoporosis?

A. Raloxifene
B. Alendronate
C. Calcitonin
D. Denosumab

Q258. Which antihistamine is commonly used for motion sickness prevention?

A. Loratadine
B. Cetirizine
C. Diphenhydramine
D. Fexofenadine

Q259. Which vitamin is essential for normal blood clotting and synthesis of coagulation factors?

A. Vitamin A
B. Vitamin C
C. Vitamin K
D. Vitamin D

Q260. Which class of drugs is prescribed to reduce anxiety without causing significant sedation or dependence?

A. Benzodiazepines
B. Buspirone
C. Barbiturates
D. Beta-blockers

Q261. Which element must be verified on every prescription before processing?

A. Patient's insurance provider
B. Prescriber's DEA number (when applicable)
C. Patient's favorite pharmacy
D. Pharmacy manager's initials

Q262. What is the pharmacy technician's main responsibility during prescription intake?

A. Review and enter prescription data accurately
B. Counsel the patient on medication usage
C. Approve refill authorizations
D. Evaluate therapeutic alternatives

Q263. When processing an e-prescription, the technician should first:

A. Print it and store it in a file
B. Confirm prescriber credentials and patient data
C. Immediately prepare the medication
D. Skip data entry to save time

Q264. What information must appear on all prescription labels?

A. Prescriber's address
B. Patient's date of birth
C. Pharmacy's phone number
D. Directions for use

Q265. When entering a new prescription, the technician should verify the drug name and:

A. Storage temperature
B. Expiration date of stock medication
C. Dosage form and strength
D. Manufacturer name

Q266. Why must technicians check for duplicate therapies before processing?

A. To ensure the patient is not overcharged
B. To prevent patients from taking the same drug twice under different names
C. To promote better insurance coverage
D. To speed up workflow

Q267. Which of the following must be verified when filling a controlled substance prescription?

A. Patient's social security number
B. Number of authorized refills
C. Patient's insurance policy
D. Copayment amount

Q268. Which step occurs immediately before the pharmacist's final check?

A. Label generation
B. Counseling the patient
C. Counting and packaging medication
D. Billing insurance

Q269. A technician receives a prescription with unclear handwriting. What should they do?

A. Guess the medication name
B. Ask another technician for input
C. Notify the pharmacist immediately
D. Call the prescriber without permission

Q270. What is the technician's responsibility in preventing look-alike/sound-alike drug errors?

A. Counseling the patient on differences
B. Storing similar drugs far apart and double-checking labels
C. Recommending brand-name drugs instead
D. Ignoring label warnings for efficiency

Q271. When processing a refill request, the technician must first:

A. Verify prescriber approval if refills have expired
B. Automatically refill the medication
C. Substitute a generic drug
D. Process the refill immediately

Q272. What is the correct first step in sterile compounding?

A. Don sterile gloves
B. Wash and disinfect hands and arms
C. Wipe vials with alcohol after compounding
D. Label the compounded product

Q273. A prescription label must include which of the following?

A. Patient's allergies
B. Medication name, strength, and dosage directions
C. Pharmacy manager's license number
D. Date of manufacturer production

Q274. What must be done if a technician discovers a medication recall affecting stock drugs?

A. Dispense remaining stock first
B. Call the manufacturer directly
C. Continue using them until the replacement arrives

D. Remove recalled drugs and notify the pharmacist

Q275. Which tool assists in detecting possible drug interactions during prescription entry?

A. Inventory management system
B. Drug utilization review (DUR) alerts
C. Stock rotation software
D. Patient loyalty program

Q276. What is the correct procedure for compounding hazardous drugs?

A. Work in a negative-pressure room using protective equipment
B. Compound them in open air for ventilation
C. Use bare hands for precision
D. Store them with non-hazardous drugs

Q277. Before a compounded sterile product (CSP) can be dispensed, it must:

A. Be verified by another technician
B. Undergo visual inspection for particulates and clarity
C. Be stored for 24 hours before use
D. Be labeled only with initials

Q278. A pharmacy technician preparing a sterile IV admixture should always:

A. Work in a horizontal laminar airflow hood
B. Wear a mask only when instructed
C. Touch vial stoppers without cleaning them
D. Face away from the airflow

Q279. What is the correct protocol when entering prescription data into the computer?

A. Skip patient verification to save time
B. Enter only drug name and skip directions
C. Verify all prescription details match the original order
D. Rely on previous records for dosage

Q280. What is the technician's responsibility in label verification?

A. Ensure label matches prescription details exactly
B. Approve refills automatically
C. Edit drug warnings without pharmacist review
D. Shorten directions to fit label space

Q281. When processing a controlled substance prescription, the technician should verify:

A. The prescriber's DEA number and prescription date
B. The patient's favorite pharmacy location
C. The drug's manufacturer
D. The patient's insurance copay

Q282. What must a pharmacy technician confirm before labeling a reconstituted antibiotic?

A. Patient's age
B. Beyond-use date and storage requirements
C. Drug manufacturer's contact
D. Patient's insurance coverage

Q283. A technician notices the NDC on a drug label does not match the bottle. What should they do?

A. Dispense it anyway if it's the same drug name
B. Notify the pharmacist immediately
C. Replace the label without checking
D. Ignore it since it's a minor issue

Q284. Which document provides instructions on handling chemical spills in the pharmacy?

A. DEA Form 222

B. Controlled Substance Log
C. Medication Guide
D. Material Safety Data Sheet (MSDS)

Q285. When should a technician use a tall-man lettering system?

A. For medications with long names
B. For look-alike or sound-alike drug names
C. For over-the-counter products only
D. For patient education materials

Q286. When receiving a new prescription, the pharmacy technician should always:

A. Confirm the prescription's authenticity and completeness
B. Call the patient for medical history
C. File the prescription without verification
D. Process the refill automatically

Q287. When compounding a non-sterile product, what must the technician verify first?

A. Prescription authenticity and formula accuracy
B. Packaging type
C. The patient's allergies
D. The product's cost

Q288. What must be checked before dispensing a medication stored in the refrigerator?

A. The color of the bottle cap
B. The medication's temperature and expiration date
C. The pharmacy technician's initials
D. The patient's co-pay amount

Q289. What is the technician's main goal during the final product preparation stage?

A. To ensure all quantities and labels match the prescription
B. To approve the medication for patient counseling
C. To verify clinical appropriateness
D. To collect payment before dispensing

Q290. What should a technician do if a prescription is missing the dosage?

A. Estimate the dosage from previous prescriptions
B. Ask the patient what dosage they prefer
C. Hold the prescription and notify the pharmacist
D. Dispense the lowest available dose

Q291. When processing a prescription for a Schedule II controlled substance, which action must be taken?

A. Allow one automatic refill
B. Require a new, written prescription for each fill
C. Dispense without pharmacist review
D. Accept a fax copy for all cases

Q292. Which step ensures accuracy during data entry of a prescription?

A. Skipping patient verification
B. Confirming patient, drug, and prescriber details before saving
C. Bypassing insurance entry to save time
D. Editing directions for brevity

Q293. Before mixing ingredients for a compound, what must the technician confirm?

A. The proper ingredients and their quantities per formula
B. The batch number of the product
C. The drug manufacturer's details

D. The expiration date of the final product

Q294. What is the purpose of using auxiliary labels on prescription bottles?

A. To replace the pharmacist's counseling
B. To provide warnings and usage reminders
C. To display the pharmacy's promotional information
D. To indicate the manufacturer's name

Q295. What should a pharmacy technician do when handling high-alert medications?

A. Label and store them separately with clear warnings
B. Dispense them quickly to reduce waiting time
C. Ignore label differences to save space
D. Handle them the same as regular medications

Q296. During prescription verification, which detail should be checked first?

A. Pharmacy location
B. Patient's insurance number
C. Drug name and strength
D. Prescription file number

Q297. When receiving a faxed prescription, what is the technician required to do?

A. Process it without review
B. Call the patient to confirm
C. File it without pharmacist approval
D. Verify the prescriber's signature and fax authenticity

Q298. A pharmacy technician must document a partial fill for which class of medication?

A. Over-the-counter drugs
B. Schedule II controlled substances
C. Herbal supplements
D. Schedule V medications

Q299. What should a pharmacy technician confirm before dispensing repackaged medications?

A. The batch number and beyond-use date
B. The manufacturer's country
C. The patient's birth date
D. The pharmacy's license number

Q300. Which type of prescription requires immediate attention by the pharmacist?

A. A refill request for an over-the-counter product
B. A new prescription with a potential drug interaction alert
C. A request for medical records
D. A prescription with no patient address

Answer keys and Explanations (201-300)

Q201. Answer: C

Explanation: Tricyclic antidepressants (TCAs) like amitriptyline inhibit reuptake of serotonin and norepinephrine, improving mood and relieving depression. They are effective but associated with significant side effects such as anticholinergic symptoms, orthostatic hypotension, and cardiac toxicity in overdose. TCAs are now second-line due to these risks, replaced by SSRIs and SNRIs for safety and better tolerability.

Q202. Answer: B

Explanation: Albuterol is a short-acting beta-2 agonist (SABA) used for quick relief of bronchospasm in asthma and COPD. It acts within minutes to relax bronchial smooth muscle, improving airflow and relieving wheezing. Overuse may lead to tachycardia and decreased effectiveness. Long-term control requires anti-inflammatory therapy such as inhaled corticosteroids, not SABAs alone.

Q203. Answer: A

Explanation: Metformin lowers blood glucose by reducing hepatic gluconeogenesis and increasing insulin sensitivity in peripheral tissues. It does not stimulate insulin release, so the risk of hypoglycemia is minimal. It is first-line therapy for type 2 diabetes due to its efficacy, safety, and possible cardiovascular benefits. Gastrointestinal upset is the most common side effect, and renal function must be monitored.

Q204. Answer: B

Explanation: Thiazide diuretics increase sodium and chloride excretion while promoting potassium loss in the distal tubule, leading to hypokalemia. They are often combined with potassium-sparing agents to balance electrolytes. Monitoring serum potassium is essential to prevent arrhythmias. Thiazides can also increase calcium reabsorption, differentiating them from loop diuretics, which typically cause both potassium and calcium losses.

Q205. Answer: B

Explanation: Fluoroquinolones, such as ciprofloxacin and levofloxacin, have FDA black box warnings for risks of tendon rupture, peripheral neuropathy, and CNS effects. They should be reserved for serious infections where benefits outweigh risks. Patients, especially the elderly or those on corticosteroids, should be advised to report musculoskeletal pain or weakness promptly to prevent irreversible injury.

Q206. Answer: C

Explanation: Opioids like oxycodone decrease gastrointestinal motility by binding to mu-opioid receptors in the gut, leading to constipation. Prophylactic use of stool softeners or laxatives is often recommended. Other side effects include sedation, respiratory depression, and nausea. Tolerance and dependence can develop with chronic use, requiring careful dose management and patient education.

Q207. Answer: B

Explanation: Glipizide is a sulfonylurea that stimulates pancreatic beta cells to secrete insulin, lowering blood glucose levels in type 2 diabetes. It carries a risk of hypoglycemia and weight gain, particularly in elderly patients or those with irregular meals. Unlike metformin, glipizide directly enhances insulin secretion, making dietary consistency and glucose monitoring essential to maintain safe glycemic control.

Q208. Answer: A

Explanation: Parkinson's disease involves degeneration of dopaminergic neurons in the substantia nigra, causing dopamine deficiency in the basal ganglia. This imbalance between dopamine and acetylcholine results in tremors, rigidity, and bradykinesia. Treatment aims to restore dopamine levels (levodopa/carbidopa) or mimic its effects with agonists, while sometimes using anticholinergic drugs to rebalance neurotransmitter activity.

Q209. Answer: B

Explanation: Enoxaparin, a low molecular weight heparin (LMWH), enhances antithrombin activity, inhibiting factor Xa and preventing clot formation. It is administered subcutaneously for prophylaxis and treatment of venous thromboembolism. Compared to unfractionated heparin, it provides predictable anticoagulation and does not require frequent laboratory monitoring. Renal function assessment is important to adjust dosing and avoid accumulation.

Q210. Answer: C

Explanation: Proton pump inhibitors (PPIs) like pantoprazole irreversibly block the H+/K+ ATPase enzyme on gastric parietal cells, suppressing final acid secretion regardless of stimulus. They are first-line agents for GERD, peptic ulcer disease, and Zollinger-Ellison syndrome. Prolonged therapy should be periodically reviewed due to potential risks such as vitamin B12 deficiency, fractures, and infections.

Q211. Answer: B

Explanation: SSRIs, such as escitalopram and sertraline, are preferred first-line therapies for generalized anxiety disorder due to efficacy and safety for long-term use. They enhance serotonergic transmission and reduce anxiety symptoms gradually over weeks. Benzodiazepines are reserved for short-term or acute relief due to dependence risk, while antipsychotics and MAOIs are not typically indicated for GAD.

Q212. Answer: B

Explanation: The annual influenza vaccine protects against circulating flu virus strains that mutate each season. It is recommended for nearly all adults, especially those with chronic conditions or weakened immunity. Inactivated and recombinant vaccines are standard, while live intranasal forms are reserved for certain populations. Yearly vaccination reduces complications and transmission rates across communities.

Q213. Answer: A

Explanation: Raloxifene acts as an estrogen agonist on bone and lipid metabolism but as an antagonist on uterine and breast tissue, preserving bone mineral density while reducing breast cancer risk. It is used in postmenopausal women for osteoporosis prevention. Unlike bisphosphonates, it does not require special administration instructions, but it carries a risk of venous thromboembolism.

Q214. Answer: A

Explanation: Naloxone is a pure opioid antagonist that competitively binds to opioid receptors, rapidly reversing respiratory depression and CNS depression in overdose cases. It acts within minutes when administered intranasally or intravenously. Because its half-life is shorter than most opioids, repeat doses or continuous infusion may be required. Education on its availability and emergency use is vital.

Q215. Answer: C

Explanation: ARBs such as losartan block angiotensin II from binding to AT1 receptors, preventing vasoconstriction and aldosterone release. This reduces afterload and fluid retention, improving heart failure symptoms and blood pressure control. They provide an alternative for patients intolerant to ACE inhibitor–induced cough. Monitoring renal function and potassium levels is necessary to avoid hyperkalemia.

Q216. Answer: A

Explanation: Benzodiazepines potentiate GABA-A receptor activity, increasing chloride ion influx and neuronal hyperpolarization, producing anxiolytic, sedative, and anticonvulsant effects. Lorazepam is commonly used for anxiety and acute seizure management. Dependence and tolerance can develop with prolonged use, so short-term therapy and gradual tapering are advised. They should not be combined with alcohol or CNS depressants.

Q217. Answer: B

Explanation: Second-generation antipsychotics such as risperidone and quetiapine antagonize both dopamine D2 and serotonin 5-HT2A receptors, balancing efficacy with fewer extrapyramidal symptoms (EPS). They remain preferred for schizophrenia and bipolar disorder. However, metabolic side effects including weight gain and glucose intolerance are common, requiring regular monitoring of metabolic parameters during therapy.

Q218. Answer: B

Explanation: Acetaminophen is a widely used analgesic and antipyretic with minimal anti-inflammatory effect. In overdose, it saturates normal metabolism pathways, leading to accumulation of hepatotoxic metabolites (NAPQI) that cause acute liver failure. Prompt administration of N-acetylcysteine acts as an antidote. Patients should avoid combining acetaminophen-containing products to prevent unintentional overdose.

Q219. Answer: A

Explanation: Levothyroxine is synthetic T4 that restores normal thyroid hormone levels in hypothyroidism, supporting metabolism and energy regulation. It should be taken on an empty stomach for optimal absorption. Overreplacement may cause symptoms of hyperthyroidism, so TSH monitoring guides dosing. Antithyroid agents like methimazole and propylthiouracil are used for hyperthyroid conditions, not deficiency states.

Q220. Answer: A

Explanation: Fibrates such as gemfibrozil activate peroxisome proliferator–activated receptor-alpha (PPAR-α), enhancing lipid metabolism and reducing triglyceride levels. They are beneficial for patients with hypertriglyceridemia or mixed dyslipidemia, especially when statins are not tolerated. Combination therapy increases myopathy risk, so monitoring for muscle pain and liver enzyme changes is advised during concurrent use.

Q221. Answer: B

Explanation: NSAIDs inhibit cyclooxygenase (COX) enzymes, decreasing prostaglandin production and thereby reducing pain, fever, and inflammation. Common agents include ibuprofen and naproxen. Chronic or high-dose use can cause gastrointestinal irritation, renal impairment, or cardiovascular risks. Unlike corticosteroids, NSAIDs act peripherally without immune suppression, making them suitable for short-term management of mild-to-moderate inflammatory conditions.

Q222. Answer: D

Explanation: Omeprazole, a proton pump inhibitor, suppresses gastric acid secretion by blocking the H^+/K^+ ATPase enzyme in stomach parietal cells. It promotes healing of erosive esophagitis and alleviates GERD symptoms. Long-term therapy should be monitored for nutrient malabsorption risks such as vitamin B12 deficiency. Lisinopril, loratadine, and metformin treat unrelated conditions and are not indicated for GERD.

Q223. Answer: B

Explanation: ARBs, such as losartan and valsartan, block angiotensin II from binding to AT1 receptors on blood vessels and adrenal glands. This prevents vasoconstriction and aldosterone-mediated fluid retention, resulting in lower blood pressure and reduced cardiac workload. They are alternatives for patients intolerant to ACE inhibitors due to cough, with similar benefits for heart failure and hypertension management.

Q224. Answer: B

Explanation: Tetracyclines bind to calcium in developing teeth and bones, leading to permanent discoloration and enamel hypoplasia when used in children under eight years. They are contraindicated during pregnancy and early childhood. Alternatives such as amoxicillin or cephalexin are safer. Tetracyclines remain valuable for acne, Lyme disease, and atypical infections in appropriate age groups.

Q225. Answer: C

Explanation: Ezetimibe selectively blocks the Niemann-Pick C1-like 1 (NPC1L1) transporter in the small intestine, reducing dietary and biliary cholesterol absorption. It effectively lowers LDL levels and is often used with statins for additive lipid control. Unlike fibrates or bile acid sequestrants, ezetimibe has minimal gastrointestinal effects and provides a well-tolerated option for hypercholesterolemia management.

Q226. Answer: A

Explanation: Valproic acid enhances GABA activity and stabilizes neuronal membranes, making it effective for seizure control and bipolar mood stabilization. It is frequently used as an alternative or adjunct to lithium. Monitoring liver function and platelets is crucial due to hepatotoxicity and thrombocytopenia risks. Common side effects include tremor, weight gain, and gastrointestinal discomfort.

Q227. Answer: C

Explanation: Loratadine is a second-generation antihistamine that selectively blocks peripheral H1 receptors without significant central nervous system penetration, minimizing drowsiness. It is used for allergic rhinitis and urticaria. Diphenhydramine and hydroxyzine, first-generation antihistamines, readily cross the blood-brain barrier, causing sedation. Cetirizine is slightly more sedating but similarly effective for allergy management.

Q228. Answer: B

Explanation: Antifungal agents such as terbinafine and fluconazole target ergosterol synthesis or function in fungal cell membranes, compromising integrity and leading to cell death. Topical or oral formulations are chosen based on infection location and severity. They differ from antibiotics that target bacteria and antivirals used for viral infections, ensuring selective activity against fungal pathogens.

Q229. Answer: A

Explanation: Acarbose delays carbohydrate digestion and absorption in the small intestine by inhibiting alpha-glucosidase enzymes, thereby lowering postprandial glucose spikes. It does not stimulate insulin release and carries a low hypoglycemia risk when used alone. Gastrointestinal side effects such as flatulence and diarrhea are common due to undigested carbohydrates reaching the colon.

Q230. Answer: A

Explanation: Allopurinol inhibits xanthine oxidase, reducing the production of uric acid and preventing gout flare-ups. It is indicated for chronic gout prophylaxis, not acute attacks. During initiation, colchicine or NSAIDs may be co-prescribed to prevent paradoxical flares. Regular monitoring of renal function and uric acid levels ensures effectiveness and safety in long-term management.

Q231. Answer: B

Explanation: Clozapine is a second-generation antipsychotic highly effective for treatment-resistant schizophrenia but can cause agranulocytosis, a potentially life-threatening drop in white blood cells. Regular monitoring of absolute neutrophil count (ANC) is mandatory. While it carries metabolic side effects similar to other atypicals, its superior efficacy justifies use under strict blood safety programs.

Q232. Answer: C

Explanation: Amlodipine is a dihydropyridine calcium channel blocker that relaxes vascular smooth muscle, decreasing peripheral resistance and blood pressure. It is used in hypertension and chronic angina. Unlike non-dihydropyridines, it minimally affects heart rate or contractility. Common adverse effects include peripheral edema, flushing, and headache, typically dose-related and managed through titration.

Q233. Answer: B

Explanation: Nitroglycerin acts as a vasodilator by releasing nitric oxide, relaxing vascular smooth muscle and reducing myocardial oxygen demand. It rapidly alleviates angina pectoris caused by myocardial ischemia. Sublingual formulations offer quick relief, while transdermal patches provide prevention. Patients should sit or lie down during use to prevent dizziness or hypotension.

Q234. Answer: A

Explanation: Ciprofloxacin, a fluoroquinolone antibiotic, is effective against Gram-negative bacteria commonly responsible for urinary tract infections. It inhibits bacterial DNA gyrase, preventing DNA replication. Though effective, its use should be limited to confirmed infections due to resistance risk and serious adverse effects like tendon injury. Alternative agents may be preferred for uncomplicated UTIs when possible.

Q235. Answer: B

Explanation: Montelukast is a leukotriene receptor antagonist that reduces airway inflammation and prevents bronchoconstriction. It is used for chronic asthma maintenance and allergic rhinitis, not acute attacks. Administered orally, it complements inhaled corticosteroids or bronchodilators. Side effects are generally mild, but rare neuropsychiatric symptoms warrant patient monitoring during long-term use.

Q236. Answer: B

Explanation: Omeprazole, available OTC, inhibits gastric acid secretion via irreversible inhibition of the proton pump (H+/K+ ATPase) in parietal cells. It provides long-lasting relief from frequent heartburn when taken daily. It is not intended for immediate relief; antacids serve that purpose. Long-term PPI use should be monitored for nutrient deficiencies and rebound acid hypersecretion.

Q237. Answer: A

Explanation: Spironolactone antagonizes aldosterone receptors in the distal nephron, promoting sodium and water excretion while conserving potassium. It is useful in hypertension, heart failure, and hyperaldosteronism. Monitoring potassium and renal function is essential to prevent hyperkalemia. Combining it with thiazide or loop diuretics provides balanced diuretic and antihypertensive effects while minimizing potassium loss.

Q238. Answer: C

Explanation: Insulin glargine is a long-acting basal insulin analogue with steady, peakless absorption over approximately 24 hours, maintaining fasting blood glucose levels. It is typically administered once daily, separate from mealtime insulin. Proper injection technique and rotation of sites prevent lipodystrophy. Regular glucose monitoring ensures dose accuracy and minimizes hypoglycemia risk.

Q239. Answer: A

Explanation: Cyclobenzaprine acts on the central nervous system to reduce muscle spasm without direct muscle effects. It is prescribed for short-term relief of acute musculoskeletal pain. Sedation and dizziness are common, requiring caution with activities requiring alertness. It should be avoided in combination with alcohol or CNS depressants and used only for limited durations to prevent dependence.

Q240. Answer: B

Explanation: Lisinopril is an ACE inhibitor that prevents the conversion of angiotensin I to angiotensin II, resulting in vasodilation and decreased aldosterone secretion. It lowers blood pressure and improves heart failure outcomes. Patients may experience a dry cough due to bradykinin accumulation. Renal function and potassium levels should be monitored to avoid adverse effects like hyperkalemia or renal impairment.

Q241. Answer: A

Explanation: Oral vancomycin is the first-line treatment for C. difficile infections because it stays in the gastrointestinal tract to inhibit bacterial cell wall synthesis without systemic absorption. It effectively eliminates toxin-producing bacteria while minimizing further microbiota disruption. Intravenous vancomycin is not effective for this condition since it does not reach adequate concentrations in the intestinal lumen.

Q242. Answer: B

Explanation: Cardiac glycosides like digoxin inhibit the sodium-potassium ATPase pump, increasing intracellular calcium and enhancing myocardial contractility. This improves cardiac output in heart failure and controls ventricular response in atrial fibrillation. Toxicity can cause visual disturbances and arrhythmias, so serum levels and electrolytes must be closely monitored, especially in patients with renal impairment.

Q243. Answer: D

Explanation: The HPV vaccine provides immunity against high-risk human papillomavirus strains responsible for cervical, anal, and other genital cancers. It is recommended for both males and females, ideally before sexual activity begins. Administered in a two- or three-dose series, the vaccine effectively reduces HPV infection prevalence and subsequent cancer risk through robust immunologic protection.

Q244. Answer: B

Explanation: Naltrexone is a long-acting opioid receptor antagonist used to maintain abstinence in opioid or alcohol dependence. Unlike naloxone, it is not for acute overdose reversal but for relapse prevention.

It blocks euphoric effects of opioids, helping motivated patients sustain recovery. Oral and extended-release injectable forms support compliance under structured addiction treatment programs.

Q245. Answer: B

Explanation: Formoterol is a long-acting beta-2 agonist (LABA) that provides bronchodilation for up to 12 hours by relaxing bronchial smooth muscle. It is used in combination with inhaled corticosteroids for maintenance therapy in asthma and COPD, not for acute symptom relief. Proper use prevents exacerbations, but LABAs should always be combined with anti-inflammatory agents to avoid monotherapy-related risks.

Q246. Answer: B

Explanation: Eradication of H. pylori infection typically involves combination therapy of antibiotics such as clarithromycin or amoxicillin with a proton pump inhibitor (PPI) to reduce acid secretion. This dual or triple therapy promotes ulcer healing and prevents recurrence. Using antacids or H2 blockers alone provides symptom relief but does not eliminate the bacterial cause of ulcers.

Q247. Answer: B

Explanation: Canagliflozin is an SGLT2 inhibitor that lowers blood glucose by increasing urinary glucose excretion through inhibition of sodium-glucose co-transporters in the proximal renal tubules. It also provides cardiovascular and renal benefits. Side effects include dehydration, genital infections, and rare cases of diabetic ketoacidosis. Adequate hydration and patient monitoring reduce potential complications.

Q248. Answer: C

Explanation: Midazolam is a short-acting benzodiazepine that enhances GABA-mediated neuronal inhibition, producing sedation, amnesia, and anxiolysis before medical procedures. Its rapid onset and short duration make it ideal for conscious sedation. Careful monitoring of respiratory function is essential due to potential respiratory depression, particularly when combined with other sedatives or opioids.

Q249. Answer: B

Explanation: Metoclopramide blocks dopamine receptors in the chemoreceptor trigger zone and enhances gastric motility, making it effective for nausea, vomiting, and gastroparesis. It carries a risk of extrapyramidal symptoms with long-term use due to dopamine blockade. Unlike ondansetron, which targets serotonin receptors, metoclopramide also improves gastric emptying in patients with diabetic gastroparesis.

Q250. Answer: A

Explanation: Vitamin B12 deficiency, often due to intrinsic factor absence or malabsorption, causes pernicious anemia characterized by megaloblastic changes and neurologic symptoms. Replacement therapy is typically administered via intramuscular injection or high-dose oral supplements. Early recognition and treatment prevent irreversible neuropathy and cognitive impairment associated with prolonged deficiency.

Q251. Answer: B

Explanation: Antihypertensive medications, including ACE inhibitors, ARBs, calcium channel blockers, beta-blockers, and diuretics, reduce blood pressure to prevent cardiovascular events like stroke and myocardial infarction. Therapy is individualized based on comorbidities and response. Lifestyle modification complements drug therapy for optimal control and long-term health outcomes.

Q252. Answer: C

Explanation: Aripiprazole acts as a partial dopamine agonist with minimal effect on weight and glucose metabolism, lowering the risk of metabolic syndrome compared to other atypical antipsychotics. It is effective for schizophrenia, bipolar disorder, and adjunctive therapy in depression. Patients still require periodic monitoring for EPS, akathisia, and general metabolic health.

Q253. Answer: A

Explanation: Phenytoin stabilizes neuronal membranes by modulating sodium channels but has a narrow therapeutic range (10–20 mcg/mL). Regular blood level monitoring prevents toxicity, which can manifest as nystagmus, ataxia, and gingival hyperplasia. Individual metabolism variability necessitates careful dose adjustment to maintain safe and effective concentrations.

Q254. Answer: A

Explanation: Tamsulosin selectively blocks alpha-1A adrenergic receptors in prostate and bladder neck smooth muscle, relaxing these tissues and improving urine flow in BPH. It does not significantly affect blood pressure. Orthostatic hypotension and dizziness may occur initially. Finasteride, a 5-alpha-reductase inhibitor, reduces prostate size but acts more slowly than tamsulosin.

Q255. Answer: D

Explanation: Corticosteroids inhibit phospholipase A2, blocking the release of arachidonic acid and thus preventing both prostaglandin and leukotriene synthesis. This broad anti-inflammatory action makes them effective for asthma, autoimmune disorders, and severe allergic reactions. Long-term use requires monitoring for adverse effects like osteoporosis, hyperglycemia, and adrenal suppression.

Q256. Answer: B

Explanation: Acetylcysteine breaks disulfide bonds in mucus proteins, decreasing viscosity and improving expectoration in conditions like chronic bronchitis or cystic fibrosis. It can be administered via nebulization or orally as an antidote for acetaminophen toxicity. When inhaled, it may cause bronchospasm; concurrent bronchodilator use minimizes this risk during therapy.

Q257. Answer: B

Explanation: Alendronate is a bisphosphonate that inhibits osteoclast-mediated bone resorption, increasing bone mineral density and reducing fracture risk. It must be taken with water on an empty stomach, with patients remaining upright for at least 30 minutes to prevent esophageal irritation. It is first-line therapy for osteoporosis in postmenopausal women and men.

Q258. Answer: C

Explanation: Diphenhydramine, a first-generation antihistamine, blocks H1 receptors and also possesses anticholinergic properties that reduce vestibular stimulation, preventing motion sickness and vertigo. It is sedating, so patients should avoid operating machinery. Non-sedating antihistamines like loratadine or fexofenadine are ineffective for motion sickness prevention due to limited central nervous system penetration.

Q259. Answer: C

Explanation: Vitamin K is required for hepatic synthesis of clotting factors II, VII, IX, and X. Deficiency leads to prolonged bleeding and bruising. It is administered to newborns at birth to prevent hemorrhagic disease and used to reverse warfarin's anticoagulant effects. Dietary sources include leafy greens, and deficiency can arise from malabsorption or prolonged antibiotic use.

Q260. Answer: B

Explanation: Buspirone is an anxiolytic that acts as a serotonin 5-HT1A receptor partial agonist, providing relief from generalized anxiety without sedation or dependence risk. It lacks anticonvulsant or muscle-relaxant properties and requires several weeks for full effect. Its favorable safety profile makes it suitable for long-term anxiety management compared to benzodiazepines.

Q261. Answer: B

Explanation: The prescriber's DEA number must be verified on every prescription involving controlled substances. This number ensures the prescription's legality and confirms that the prescriber is authorized to prescribe such medications. Technicians help the pharmacist verify this to prevent fraud, maintain regulatory compliance, and ensure safe dispensing of controlled medications in accordance with DEA and state requirements.

Q262. Answer: A

Explanation: During prescription intake, pharmacy technicians must accurately review and enter prescription data, including patient details, drug name, strength, dosage, and directions. This ensures the pharmacist can verify the information correctly before dispensing. Accuracy at this step prevents medication errors, ensures compliance with regulations, and promotes safe patient care through reliable documentation.

Q263. Answer: B

Explanation: For e-prescriptions, confirming prescriber credentials and verifying patient data ensures authenticity and accuracy before processing. This prevents errors and fraudulent prescriptions. It also ensures that the medication is dispensed only under valid authorization. Proper verification supports compliance with DEA e-prescribing regulations and ensures the patient's safety by preventing dispensing of incorrect or unauthorized medications.

Q264. Answer: D

Explanation: Directions for use are a mandatory component on all prescription labels because they guide patients on how to take their medications safely and effectively. Clear instructions reduce the risk of misuse, underdosing, or overdosing. This information ensures adherence to therapy, supports patient safety, and meets state and federal labeling regulations.

Q265. Answer: C

Explanation: Verifying the drug's dosage form and strength ensures the correct medication is dispensed as prescribed. Different forms (tablet, capsule, liquid) or strengths can significantly impact therapeutic outcomes. Double-checking this information minimizes medication errors and guarantees that the pharmacist reviews the correct product for verification before final dispensing.

Q266. Answer: B

Explanation: Checking for duplicate therapies prevents patients from unknowingly taking multiple versions of the same medication. Duplicate therapy can cause overdosing and adverse drug reactions. By identifying and alerting the pharmacist, the technician supports medication safety and ensures appropriate therapeutic management for each patient.

Q267. Answer: B

Explanation: Controlled substance prescriptions have strict limits on the number of authorized refills, which must be verified before dispensing. Technicians confirm this information to ensure compliance with DEA and state regulations. Unauthorized refills can result in legal violations and patient safety risks, making refill verification essential for lawful and safe medication handling.

Q268. Answer: C

Explanation: Counting and packaging the medication occurs just before the pharmacist's final verification. The technician must ensure accuracy in dosage, labeling, and container choice. This step ensures that when the pharmacist performs the final check, all elements of the prescription are ready and correct for dispensing. It's a crucial accuracy checkpoint in the dispensing workflow.

Q269. Answer: C

Explanation: If a prescription is unclear, the technician must notify the pharmacist immediately. Only the pharmacist can contact the prescriber to clarify prescription details. This ensures medication accuracy and prevents dispensing errors caused by misinterpretation. The technician's role is to recognize potential confusion and escalate appropriately, ensuring compliance with pharmacy procedures.

Q270. Answer: B

Explanation: Look-alike/sound-alike medications pose a significant safety risk. Technicians must store similar drugs separately and verify labels during dispensing. This minimizes confusion and ensures accurate selection. Implementing these precautions supports the ISMP's best practices and helps prevent dangerous medication mix-ups that could harm patients.

Q271. Answer: A

Explanation: When refills have expired, technicians must obtain prescriber approval before processing. This ensures that the medication therapy remains appropriate and legally authorized. Dispensing without authorization violates pharmacy law and endangers patient safety. Proper verification keeps the refill process compliant and prevents unauthorized dispensing.

Q272. Answer: B
Explanation: Handwashing and disinfection are the first steps in sterile compounding to maintain aseptic conditions. This eliminates contaminants that could compromise product sterility. Adhering to USP <797> standards, this step is essential for patient safety, preventing infection, and maintaining compliance with compounding regulations.
Q273. Answer: B
Explanation: The medication name, strength, and directions for use must always appear on a prescription label to ensure the patient receives the correct product and understands how to take it safely. This information promotes accurate administration, enhances compliance, and meets state and federal labeling laws for safe pharmaceutical practice.
Q274. Answer: D
Explanation: Upon learning of a medication recall, technicians must immediately remove all affected stock and notify the pharmacist. The pharmacist will determine next steps, such as returning the product or informing patients. Quick removal ensures that no affected medications reach patients, maintaining safety and regulatory compliance.
Q275. Answer: B
Explanation: Drug utilization review (DUR) alerts automatically identify potential drug interactions, allergies, or contraindications during prescription entry. These alerts allow the technician to flag issues for the pharmacist's evaluation, enhancing medication safety. DUR systems are vital safeguards in modern pharmacy workflows that help prevent adverse drug events and improve overall patient care.
Q276. Answer: A
Explanation: Hazardous drugs must be compounded in a negative-pressure room using protective equipment like gloves, gowns, and respirators. This environment prevents contamination and exposure, ensuring safety for both patients and pharmacy staff. Adherence to USP <800> standards maintains compliance and minimizes risk associated with handling toxic medications.
Q277. Answer: B
Explanation: All compounded sterile products must undergo a visual inspection for particulates, clarity, and container integrity before dispensing. This ensures the product meets sterility and quality standards per USP <797>. Detecting contamination or defects protects patients from potential infections or dosing inaccuracies and maintains sterile compounding integrity.
Q278. Answer: A
Explanation: Sterile IV admixtures must be prepared in a horizontal laminar airflow hood, where filtered air maintains sterility. The technician works within the airflow area to prevent contamination. Adhering to aseptic technique ensures product safety and complies with USP <797> requirements for sterile compounding environments.
Q279. Answer: C
Explanation: During data entry, technicians must ensure all prescription details—patient name, drug name, strength, quantity, and directions—match the original order exactly. Accurate data entry prevents medication errors, supports pharmacist verification, and ensures safe dispensing. Careful entry safeguards against transcription errors that could lead to adverse outcomes.
Q280. Answer: A
Explanation: The technician must ensure that every printed label matches the prescription exactly in drug name, dosage, strength, and directions. Label verification prevents dispensing errors and ensures that the patient receives the correct instructions. Accuracy at this stage is critical before pharmacist final review and contributes to patient safety and compliance.
Q281. Answer: A
Explanation: Verifying the prescriber's DEA number and prescription date ensures the controlled substance prescription is valid and compliant with DEA regulations. The date confirms that it falls within

the allowable timeframe for dispensing. These verifications help prevent misuse and ensure legal compliance when handling controlled medications.

Q282. Answer: B

Explanation: Before labeling reconstituted antibiotics, technicians must verify the beyond-use date (BUD) and proper storage conditions, such as refrigeration. This ensures medication stability and effectiveness until the BUD expires. Accurate labeling provides critical information for patient safety and compliance with USP <795> and manufacturer guidelines.

Q283. Answer: B

Explanation: If the National Drug Code (NDC) number on the label doesn't match the bottle, the technician must notify the pharmacist immediately. The NDC identifies the drug manufacturer, strength, and form—any mismatch could signal a serious dispensing error. Reporting ensures correction before dispensing, maintaining accuracy and patient safety.

Q284. Answer: D

Explanation: The Material Safety Data Sheet (MSDS) provides specific guidance on how to safely handle, contain, and clean up chemical spills. It details protective measures, first-aid instructions, and disposal procedures. Technicians must know where MSDS files are stored to ensure quick, safe responses to hazardous incidents in compliance with OSHA standards.

Q285. Answer: B

Explanation: The tall-man lettering system (e.g., predniSONE vs. prednisoLONE) is used to distinguish look-alike or sound-alike drug names. This practice reduces the risk of medication selection errors by emphasizing distinct letter patterns. Technicians apply this system during labeling and storage to promote accuracy and align with ISMP safety recommendations.

Q286. Answer: A

Explanation: Authenticity and completeness are essential to ensure the prescription is valid and accurate. A technician must check that all required elements—patient information, prescriber's signature, date, and drug details—are present and legible. This prevents errors, fraud, and regulatory violations. Verification ensures that the pharmacist reviews an accurate prescription before dispensing, maintaining patient safety and compliance with pharmacy law.

Q287. Answer: A

Explanation: Verifying the prescription's authenticity and formula accuracy is the first step in non-sterile compounding. This ensures the compounded product matches the prescriber's intent and is safe for the patient. Accuracy in ingredients and concentrations prevents medication errors and supports compliance with USP <795> standards for non-sterile compounding procedures.

Q288. Answer: B

Explanation: Before dispensing refrigerated medications, the technician must verify that the medication is stored at the correct temperature and has not expired. Temperature-sensitive drugs lose potency if not properly stored. Confirming expiration and temperature ensures drug effectiveness and patient safety, complying with manufacturer storage guidelines and regulatory standards for pharmaceutical integrity.

Q289. Answer: A

Explanation: During final product preparation, the technician must ensure the medication quantity, strength, and label information match the prescription exactly. This step prevents dispensing errors before the pharmacist's verification. Attention to detail here ensures that the pharmacist reviews a complete, accurate prescription for final check, maintaining safety and workflow efficiency.

Q290. Answer: C

Explanation: When dosage information is missing, the technician must hold the prescription and notify the pharmacist immediately. Only the pharmacist can contact the prescriber to verify and correct missing or unclear information. This ensures medication accuracy and legality, preventing unsafe or incorrect dosing that could harm the patient.

Q291. Answer: B
Explanation: Schedule II controlled substances require a new, written prescription for each fill and cannot be refilled automatically. This strict control prevents misuse, diversion, and abuse of these high-risk medications. Technicians must follow DEA regulations and verify prescription authenticity before processing, ensuring compliance with federal and state laws.
Q292. Answer: B
Explanation: Confirming patient, drug, and prescriber details before saving ensures all information is correct and matches the original prescription. This reduces the risk of medication errors caused by transcription mistakes. Data entry accuracy is a critical component of safe dispensing, forming the foundation for pharmacist verification and patient safety.
Q293. Answer: A
Explanation: The technician must confirm the proper ingredients and quantities according to the compounding formula before mixing. This verification step ensures the compounded medication meets the prescribed concentration and therapeutic intent. Precise ingredient measurement maintains product quality and compliance with USP standards, ensuring the patient receives a safe and effective preparation.
Q294. Answer: B
Explanation: Auxiliary labels provide additional information, such as warnings ("May cause drowsiness") or usage instructions ("Take with food"). These labels help patients use their medications safely and properly. While they do not replace counseling, they reinforce important information and enhance patient understanding of safe medication practices, reducing the likelihood of misuse or side effects.
Q295. Answer: A
Explanation: High-alert medications, such as insulin and anticoagulants, require extra precautions. Technicians must label and store them separately with clear warnings to avoid selection and dispensing errors. Following ISMP guidelines helps prevent serious harm due to mix-ups, ensuring high-alert medications are handled with the highest level of accuracy and safety.
Q296. Answer: C
Explanation: Checking the drug name and strength first ensures the medication matches the prescriber's order exactly. This step is essential to avoid dispensing errors that could harm the patient. Verifying drug details before all else provides a foundation for accurate and safe pharmacy operations, supporting the pharmacist's final verification.
Q297. Answer: D
Explanation: Faxed prescriptions must be verified for authenticity, including the prescriber's signature and valid fax source. Technicians ensure that prescriptions are received through authorized systems and contain all required information before processing. This verification step helps prevent fraud and ensures compliance with DEA and state pharmacy regulations.
Q298. Answer: B
Explanation: Partial fills must be documented for Schedule II controlled substances, as these medications have strict regulations under the DEA. Documentation must include the amount dispensed and the remaining quantity to ensure compliance and prevent diversion. This recordkeeping ensures accountability, legality, and accurate tracking of controlled substances within the pharmacy.
Q299. Answer: A
Explanation: Before dispensing repackaged medications, the technician must verify the batch number and beyond-use date. These details ensure the medication's traceability and confirm that it remains safe and effective for use. Proper labeling and documentation of repackaged items help maintain product integrity and meet regulatory standards for quality assurance.
Q300. Answer: B
Explanation: Any prescription that triggers a potential drug interaction alert requires immediate pharmacist review. The pharmacist must assess the risk and determine whether the prescribed

combination is safe. Technicians are responsible for flagging such alerts promptly to prevent adverse drug reactions, ensuring patient safety and adherence to quality assurance protocols.
```
```

Questions (301-400)

Q301. What must be done when a medication guide is required for a prescription?

A. File it with the patient's profile
B. Attach it to the medication at the time of dispensing
C. Provide it only upon patient request
D. Keep it in the pharmacy for reference

Q302. What must be confirmed before compounding a sterile IV solution?

A. Expiration date of diluents and drug vials
B. Patient's insurance information
C. The prescriber's medical license
D. The pharmacy's accreditation number

Q303. When labeling compounded products, what must always appear on the label?

A. Pharmacist's initials only
B. Storage instructions and beyond-use date
C. Technician's certification number
D. Manufacturer's name

Q304. What must a technician do if they receive a verbal prescription over the phone?

A. Transcribe it accurately and repeat it back for confirmation
B. Record only the medication name
C. Write it down without repeating
D. Process it immediately without pharmacist review

Q305. When verifying a patient's identity before dispensing, what should the technician request?

A. Insurance card only
B. Prescription number only
C. Date of birth and address
D. Social security number

Q306. Which of the following describes proper recordkeeping for controlled substances?

A. Maintaining separate records for controlled and non-controlled drugs
B. Storing all records together for simplicity
C. Deleting records after one year
D. Keeping records in a locked drawer only

Q307. What is the technician's responsibility when a prescription error is discovered before dispensing?

A. Notify the pharmacist immediately and stop processing
B. Correct the error independently
C. Dispense the medication with a note
D. Inform the patient directly

Q308. Which label element helps identify a medication's manufacturer and formulation?

A. DEA number
B. NDC number
C. Batch code
D. Pharmacy license number

Q309. What must a technician do before dispensing an expired medication?

A. Discard or return it according to pharmacy policy
B. Offer it to patients with a discount
C. Re-label it with a new expiration date
D. Dispense it if the pharmacist approves

Q310. Which step helps prevent cross-contamination during non-sterile compounding?

A. Skipping surface disinfection to save time
B. Mixing different medications in one area
C. Handling powders and liquids simultaneously
D. Wearing gloves and cleaning equipment before and after compounding

Q311. Before dispensing, the technician must verify that the quantity in the bottle matches the prescription. Why is this step critical?
A. It ensures billing accuracy
B. It prevents dispensing errors and dosage discrepancies
C. It helps speed up workflow
D. It satisfies insurance audits

Q312. When labeling a compounded medication, the technician must always include:
A. The patient's insurance ID
B. The initials of the technician
C. The name and concentration of each active ingredient
D. The price of the compounded product

Q313. What action should a pharmacy technician take if a patient requests a generic substitution?
A. Substitute it immediately without approval
B. Confirm substitution is permitted and notify the pharmacist
C. Decline the request
D. Record it as a brand-name sale

Q314. What must the technician check before entering a refill request into the system?
A. Prescription number and remaining refills
B. Manufacturer name
C. Drug price
D. Pharmacy location

Q315. When receiving a verbal prescription from a prescriber, which detail is mandatory?
A. The patient's insurance coverage
B. The prescriber's name and DEA number (if applicable)
C. The pharmacy's contact number
D. The technician's initials

Q316. What should a pharmacy technician do if the pharmacy management system shows a drug interaction alert?
A. Dismiss it and continue
B. Override it for efficiency
C. Notify the pharmacist immediately
D. Delete the patient's profile

Q317. What is the main reason for documenting lot numbers on compounded medications?
A. To verify expiration dates
B. To ensure traceability in case of a recall
C. To record technician productivity
D. To report manufacturing costs

Q318. Which of the following actions best supports inventory control in the pharmacy?
A. Ignoring expired stock
B. Rotating inventory so older stock is used first
C. Ordering medications only when shelves are empty
D. Storing all drugs together

Q319. What is the technician's first step when preparing a new IV admixture?
A. Verify ingredients and compatibility

B. Label the final product first
C. Skip handwashing for efficiency
D. Use open-air workspace

Q320. Which documentation is required when dispensing a controlled substance?
A. Pharmacist's license
B. DEA number and dispensing record
C. Pharmacy technician's certificate
D. Manufacturer's phone number

Q321. What must the technician verify when filling a liquid medication?
A. The bottle cap color
B. The correct concentration and measuring device
C. The medication's flavor
D. The pharmacy owner's initials

Q322. A prescription label reads "Take 1 tablet q8h." What must the technician ensure?
A. The directions match prescriber's original instructions
B. The tablet color matches the reference image
C. The label font size is enlarged
D. The patient's insurance covers it

Q323. When packaging a unit dose medication, the technician must include:
A. Patient name and storage conditions
B. Drug name, strength, and expiration date
C. Pharmacist initials only
D. Manufacturer phone number

Q324. When should a pharmacy technician complete cleaning of the laminar airflow hood?
A. Once per day
B. Only when visible residue appears
C. Weekly only
D. Before each sterile compounding session and after spills

Q325. A technician notices a foreign particle in a sterile compounded solution. What should be done?
A. Filter it out and continue
B. Discard the solution and report to the pharmacist
C. Label it as non-sterile
D. Dispense after inspection

Q326. Which step ensures proper hand hygiene before sterile compounding?
A. Using an alcohol-based sanitizer only
B. Washing hands and forearms thoroughly for at least 30 seconds
C. Wearing gloves without washing hands
D. Wiping hands on a dry towel only

Q327. A pharmacy technician must document a compounding error immediately because:
A. It ensures transparency and process improvement
B. It increases productivity
C. It avoids blame
D. It allows the product to be reused

Q328. What should the technician verify on the manufacturer's medication bottle before counting?
A. NDC, drug name, and strength
B. Price and color of bottle cap
C. Pharmacist's initials
D. Insurance number

Q329. What is the main purpose of using a bar-code verification system in dispensing?
A. To improve insurance billing
B. To verify the correct drug and patient match
C. To record sales volume
D. To print medication guides
Q330. When should a technician perform double-count verification?
A. For all medications, especially controlled substances
B. Only for over-the-counter drugs
C. Only if the pharmacist is unavailable
D. Only when requested by the patient
Q331. A prescription label must include which date?
A. The patient's birth date
B. The date of dispensing
C. The date the pharmacy opened
D. The pharmacist's license issue date
Q332. Which of the following ensures sterility during the transfer of sterile solutions?
A. Avoiding contact between sterile surfaces and non-sterile objects
B. Using any gloves available
C. Blowing air across the workspace
D. Holding vials outside the airflow
Q333. What information must be recorded when a compounded batch is prepared?
A. Pharmacist's license number
B. Pharmacy manager's phone number
C. Technician name, ingredient lot numbers, and quantities used
D. Patient's insurance code
Q334. Which of the following is required before dispensing an antibiotic suspension?
A. Reconstituting it with the correct amount of diluent
B. Labeling it without reconstitution
C. Mixing it with water of any volume
D. Handing it to the patient dry
Q335. Why is it essential to include storage instructions on all medication labels?
A. To ensure drugs are stored safely and maintain potency
B. To provide marketing information
C. To satisfy insurance requirements
D. To make labels look complete
Q336. What must a technician confirm before printing a prescription label?
A. All data matches the original prescription exactly
B. The pharmacy's contact number is visible
C. The color of the label template
D. The patient's insurance plan
Q337. When handling expired controlled substances, the technician must:
A. Destroy them independently
B. Segregate and document them for pharmacist review
C. Reuse them for compounding
D. Return them to stock
Q338. Which type of prescription can legally be transferred between pharmacies?
A. Schedule II controlled substances
B. Schedule III–V controlled substances (once)

C. All controlled substances indefinitely
D. Non-controlled only with prescriber approval

Q339. Why must the technician record the expiration date on each repackaged item?
A. To maintain accurate stock rotation and prevent dispensing expired products
B. To ensure insurance claims process faster
C. To track technician productivity
D. To comply with manufacturer advertising

Q340. What is the technician's primary task during the pharmacist's final check?
A. Verify the prescriber's credentials
B. Review prescriptions for clinical appropriateness
C. Counsel patients on side effects
D. Observe and correct labeling errors before pharmacist approval

Q341. What is required when returning a controlled substance to the supplier?
A. Completion of DEA Form 222
B. Verbal notification only
C. Recording in a daily sales log
D. Fax confirmation from the supplier

Q342. Which of the following is critical in ensuring patient confidentiality during dispensing?
A. Discussing prescription details only with authorized personnel
B. Reviewing prescriptions in public areas
C. Sharing refill information with family members
D. Displaying patient names on open counters

Q343. Before dispensing, a technician should ensure the prescription label includes:
A. Pharmacy's logo and slogan
B. Patient's name, drug name, and dosage directions
C. Prescriber's personal address
D. Pharmacist's state license number

Q344. Which process ensures sterility when transferring sterile solutions?
A. Disinfecting vial stoppers with 70% isopropyl alcohol
B. Wiping stoppers with water
C. Using bare hands to minimize static
D. Holding vials outside the airflow hood

Q345. What is required on a unit-dose package label for hospital use?
A. Pharmacy phone number and technician initials
B. Drug name, strength, lot number, and expiration date
C. Drug price and prescriber's DEA number
D. Manufacturer's contact information

Q346. Which of the following ensures accuracy during manual counting?
A. Using a clean counting tray and spatula for each medication
B. Mixing similar tablets to save time
C. Counting tablets by hand without gloves
D. Leaving residue on the tray

Q347. Which of these drugs should always be handled in a biological safety cabinet?
A. Antineoplastic (chemotherapy) drugs
B. Over-the-counter antihistamines
C. Nonsteroidal anti-inflammatory drugs
D. Antibiotic tablets

Q348. What is the technician's role in third-party claim rejections?

A. Contact the prescriber directly for reimbursement
B. Change prescription details to make it payable
C. Ignore the rejection and dispense
D. Resolve billing issues and alert the pharmacist

Q349. When a prescription balance due notice appears, the technician should:
A. Dispense only after full payment
B. Inform the patient politely and process the claim again if needed
C. Cancel the prescription immediately
D. Override the system warning

Q350. What is required when a pharmacy repackages bulk medication into smaller containers?
A. New labeling with drug name, strength, lot number, and beyond-use date
B. Removing the manufacturer's label
C. Mixing medications for efficiency
D. Omitting expiration dates

Q351. What is the technician's first action when a medication recall alert appears?
A. Isolate the affected medication immediately
B. Continue dispensing until supplies run out
C. Delete the alert from the system
D. Notify patients directly

Q352. Which situation requires the use of DEA Form 106?
A. Loss or theft of controlled substances
B. Expired medication disposal
C. Medication recall notice
D. Routine inventory adjustment

Q353. What is the correct action when identifying a forged prescription?
A. Record it as a cash sale
B. Attempt to fill it discreetly
C. Notify the pharmacist immediately
D. Ignore and file the prescription

Q354. Why is label reconciliation important before pharmacist verification?
A. It ensures label information matches the prescription and product exactly
B. It confirms the pharmacy's logo is printed correctly
C. It checks patient payment details
D. It helps with advertising compliance

Q355. What must be done with hazardous waste generated from compounding?
A. Dispose of it following OSHA and EPA guidelines in labeled containers
B. Place it with regular trash
C. Flush it down the sink
D. Store it indefinitely

Q356. What is the correct procedure when a prescriber cancels a prescription?
A. Continue to fill it until confirmed
B. Delete it without record
C. Mark it as "void" and document cancellation in the patient's record
D. File it for later review

Q357. What is the technician's responsibility when preparing a controlled substance inventory?
A. Accurately count and document quantities on hand
B. Estimate quantities for speed
C. Exclude expired stock

D. Record only Schedule V drugs

Q358. Why must the technician ensure auxiliary labels are applied correctly?

A. They convey essential warnings for safe medication use

B. They improve the bottle's appearance

C. They increase sales of prescriptions

D. They replace pharmacist counseling

Q359. What is the technician's responsibility during automated dispensing system maintenance?

A. Delegate all maintenance to the pharmacist

B. Verify calibration, cleanliness, and correct drug loading

C. Ignore alerts during operation

D. Leave unused tablets in bins indefinitely

Q360. Before sending out a filled prescription, the technician should always:

A. Match the prescription label to the stock bottle used

B. Skip verification to save time

C. Staple unrelated patient materials

D. Change directions if unclear

Q361. What is the correct first step before filling any prescription?

A. Begin counting tablets

B. Prepare the medication label

C. Select the stock bottle

D. Verify patient identity and prescription validity

Q362. Why is maintaining a perpetual inventory of controlled substances important?

A. It allows continuous monitoring for discrepancies or diversion

B. It increases sales accuracy

C. It reduces paperwork requirements

D. It helps reorder non-controlled drugs

Q363. When handling cytotoxic (chemotherapy) medications, the technician must:

A. Use personal protective equipment and a biological safety cabinet

B. Wear a simple surgical mask

C. Compound them on an open countertop

D. Avoid documentation for confidentiality

Q364. What must a pharmacy technician confirm before placing a label on a container?

A. The drug name is spelled creatively for space The

B. The label is printed with the pharmacy logo

C. The label font color matches the template

D. container holds the exact medication and quantity prescribed

Q365. A pharmacy technician receives a duplicate prescription from the same provider. What should be done first?

A. Alert the pharmacist before processing

B. Fill both prescriptions to ensure supply

C. Cancel the older order

D. Contact the patient for clarification

Q366. Why must medications with a Risk Evaluation and Mitigation Strategy (REMS) be dispensed under specific procedures?

A. To ensure patient safety for high-risk medications

B. To satisfy manufacturer marketing requirements

C. To improve refill frequency

D. To bypass counseling requirements

Q367. Which of the following actions best maintains workflow accuracy during busy pharmacy hours?
A. Skipping verification steps to save time
B. Processing one prescription at a time in sequence
C. Delegating all verification to the pharmacist
D. Processing multiple patients simultaneously
Q368. What is required when compounding sterile preparations to prevent contamination?
A. Adhering to aseptic technique and using sterile equipment
B. Wearing casual attire
C. Using open containers
D. Skipping surface disinfection
Q369. Why must a pharmacy technician maintain accurate patient profiles?
A. To assist in pharmacy marketing
B. To reduce paperwork requirements
C. To help prevent drug interactions and duplicate therapy
D. To eliminate pharmacist review
Q370. Which storage condition is correct for most reconstituted antibiotic suspensions?
A. Refrigerated at 2–8°C unless otherwise specified
B. Kept at room temperature indefinitely
C. Stored near heating equipment
D. Frozen for stability
Q371. Why must all measuring devices used in compounding be calibrated regularly?
A. To ensure measurement accuracy and consistent product quality
B. To comply with cosmetic labeling standards
C. To increase compounding speed
D. To avoid replacing old equipment
Q372. Which component is mandatory on all prescription labels by federal law?
A. Directions for use and prescriber's name
B. Patient's social security number
C. Pharmacy's logo and motto
D. Technician's initials
Q373. When filling a controlled prescription, the technician must verify the DEA number using what formula?
A. Multiply all digits together
B. Add the 1st, 3rd, and 5th digits; add 2nd, 4th, and 6th digits × 2; last digit equals the DEA check digit
C. Match only the first two letters
D. Use the state license number
Q374. What step must be taken before entering a new patient into the system?
A. Verify spelling, address, and date of birth against valid ID
B. Assign a random ID number
C. Skip allergy information for speed
D. Save profile without confirmation
Q375. What must be included when preparing a compounding record?
A. The patient's insurance number
B. Only the prescriber's signature
C. Ingredients used, quantities, lot numbers, and beyond-use date
D. Pharmacist's shift schedule
Q376. What is the technician's responsibility when a prescription SIG is unclear?
A. Notify the pharmacist for clarification

B. Interpret it based on personal judgment
C. Guess używ common abbreviations
D. Proceed without confirming

Q377. Which precaution reduces light degradation of sensitive drugs?
A. Using amber or opaque containers for dispensing
B. Storing in clear bottles
C. Keeping them in direct sunlight
D. Freezing the medication

Q378. Why is documentation of refrigerator temperatures important in pharmacies?
A. It verifies prescription volume
B. It helps predict future inventory trends
C. It reduces electricity costs
D. It ensures medications are stored within safe temperature ranges

Q379. What must a technician do before using a bottle returned to stock?
A. Verify expiration date and integrity of the seal
B. Count contents blindly
C. Reuse it immediately
D. Place it in any bin

Q380. When compounding topical ointments, the technician must ensure:
A. Homogeneous mixing of ingredients
B. Application instructions are omitted
C. Ingredients are added randomly
D. The product is not labeled

Q381. What is the technician's role in ensuring accurate insurance billing?
A. Estimate copays to save time
B. Enter prescription and patient data precisely before claim submission
C. Modify claim responses
D. Skip entering diagnosis codes

Q382. Which of the following ensures accountability during controlled substance handling?
A. Double verification of every transaction and signature logs
B. Verbal confirmation only
C. Batching all entries weekly
D. Allowing one technician to manage records

Q383. Why should pharmacy work surfaces be cleaned frequently?
A. To make the workspace look tidy
B. To meet visual inspection standards
C. To prepare for audits only
D. To prevent contamination and maintain product integrity

Q384. When filling a multi-dose inhaler prescription, the technician must verify:
A. Device type, dose counter, and correct labeling
B. The patient's copay
C. The drug color only
D. Manufacturer's logo design

Q385. What must a technician ensure before dispensing reconstituted eye drops?
A. Sterility, correct dilution, and beyond-use date
B. Label readability only
C. Storage at room temperature
D. Minimal mixing

Q386. Why must a pharmacy technician record the lot number when dispensing medication?
A. To document sales for marketing
B. To help determine medication pricing
C. To trace the product in case of recalls or adverse events
D. To identify the prescribing provider
Q387. What is the technician's role during pharmacist verification?
A. Ensure the prescription is fully prepared and accurate before review
B. Approve the prescription independently
C. Change the medication based on stock
D. Skip labeling to save time
Q388. What is required before compounding an IV admixture?
A. Labeling the syringe first
B. Verification of drug compatibility and correct diluent
C. Mixing without checking orders
D. Ignoring expiration dates
Q389. Why should high-alert medications be stored separately?
A. To prevent mix-ups and accidental dispensing errors
B. To improve inventory space
C. To make them easier to find
D. To meet marketing guidelines
Q390. What should be done when a patient requests an early refill on a controlled substance?
A. Inform the pharmacist for evaluation and prescriber verification
B. Approve the refill immediately
C. Alter the date to allow early fill
D. Tell the patient to try another pharmacy
Q391. Why is label clarity essential in prescription dispensing?
A. To display marketing slogans
B. To make labels visually appealing
C. To ensure patients can read and follow dosage instructions safely
D. To avoid pharmacist verification
Q392. When reconstituting an oral suspension, the technician should:
A. Add the exact amount of diluent as indicated on the manufacturer's label
B. Use any available water source
C. Estimate the diluent volume
D. Shake before adding water
Q393. What must be done when transferring a prescription to another pharmacy?
A. Ignore the prescriber's approval
B. Send only the patient's name
C. Refill the prescription first
D. Document all transfer details, including pharmacy names and dates
Q394. What is the main purpose of beyond-use dating (BUD)?
A. To indicate the safe period for medication use after preparation
B. To record inventory delivery date
C. To schedule technician shifts
D. To determine billing cycles
Q395. What should be verified when selecting a drug from inventory?
A. Drug name, strength, and National Drug Code (NDC)
B. Color of the bottle

C. Distributor's phone number
D. Patient's insurance plan

Q396. Which practice ensures accuracy in counting tablets?
A. Counting multiple prescriptions simultaneously
B. Using a designated counting tray and verifying totals before labeling
C. Handling tablets with bare hands
D. Estimating quantities visually

Q397. Why must a technician confirm the prescriber's credentials before processing?
A. To verify authorization for prescribing specific medications
B. To check the prescriber's insurance
C. To confirm marketing preferences
D. To record for survey purposes

Q398. Which step is essential before entering prescription information into the system?
A. Reviewing the prescription for completeness and legibility
B. Entering details directly without checking
C. Asking the patient to rewrite it
D. Filing it immediately

Q399. What must be verified before dispensing a sterile compounded product?
A. Pharmacist initials
B. Product color uniformity only
C. Clarity, particulate absence, and labeling accuracy
D. Patient payment information

Q400. When preparing hazardous drugs, which engineering control must be used?
A. Biological safety cabinet or compounding aseptic containment isolator
B. Regular laminar airflow hood
C. Open countertop
D. Standard dispensing tray

Answer keys and Explanations (301-400)

Q301. Answer: B
Explanation: Medication guides are FDA-required documents that must be given to patients when dispensing certain medications, especially those with significant risks. The technician must ensure the guide is attached or provided with the prescription to educate patients on proper use and potential side effects. This ensures regulatory compliance and supports patient understanding of medication safety.
Q302. Answer: A
Explanation: Before compounding sterile IV solutions, technicians must check the expiration dates of all components, including drug vials and diluents. Using expired ingredients compromises sterility and effectiveness. Confirming this ensures product safety and compliance with USP <797> guidelines for sterile compounding practices, maintaining the integrity and efficacy of the final preparation.
Q303. Answer: B
Explanation: Every compounded product label must include storage instructions and the beyond-use date (BUD). These details guide safe handling and indicate the timeframe within which the product remains stable and effective. Proper labeling ensures compliance with compounding regulations, supports patient safety, and helps healthcare providers handle medications correctly after dispensing.
Q304. Answer: A
Explanation: When taking a verbal prescription, technicians must carefully transcribe and repeat the order back to the prescriber to ensure accuracy. This step prevents transcription errors and confirms the medication, dosage, and directions are correct. The pharmacist must always review and approve the verbal order before processing to maintain patient safety and legal compliance.
Q305. Answer: C
Explanation: Verifying the patient's date of birth and address ensures the correct patient receives the correct medication. These identifiers are reliable and reduce the risk of dispensing errors caused by similar names or duplicate profiles. This verification step is essential for maintaining accurate patient records and preventing potentially harmful mix-ups.
Q306. Answer: A
Explanation: Controlled substances must have separate records from non-controlled drugs to meet DEA requirements. This separation ensures accurate tracking, easier auditing, and compliance with federal regulations. Maintaining detailed and accessible records supports accountability, helps identify discrepancies, and prevents diversion or misuse of controlled medications within the pharmacy.
Q307. Answer: A
Explanation: If a prescription error is discovered, the technician must immediately notify the pharmacist and stop processing. The pharmacist will review and correct the issue before dispensing. This ensures patient safety, prevents medication errors, and maintains regulatory compliance by following proper reporting procedures within the pharmacy workflow.
Q308. Answer: B
Explanation: The National Drug Code (NDC) identifies the manufacturer, product, and formulation of each medication. It ensures accurate selection during dispensing and prevents substitution errors. Technicians use NDC numbers to match the prescribed drug with the correct stock, maintaining product consistency and compliance with pharmacy inventory regulations.
Q309. Answer: A
Explanation: Expired medications must never be dispensed. The technician must remove and either discard or return them according to pharmacy policy. Dispensing expired drugs violates safety regulations and may reduce therapeutic effectiveness. Proper handling ensures compliance with pharmacy law and guarantees that all dispensed medications are safe and effective.
Q310. Answer: D

Explanation: Wearing gloves and cleaning equipment before and after compounding prevents cross-contamination between substances. This ensures product purity, protects patients from unintended exposure, and meets USP <795> requirements for non-sterile compounding hygiene. Proper cleaning and personal protective equipment help maintain a safe and contaminant-free compounding environment.

Q311. Answer: B

Explanation: Verifying the quantity ensures the patient receives the correct number of doses as prescribed. Dispensing an incorrect amount can lead to underdosing or overdosing, compromising treatment effectiveness or safety. By double-checking counts and comparing against the prescription, the technician maintains accuracy, supports pharmacist verification, and upholds patient safety and regulatory compliance in the dispensing process.

Q312. Answer: C

Explanation: The label of a compounded medication must include the name and concentration of each active ingredient. This ensures proper identification, transparency, and safe administration. Including this information supports traceability and helps healthcare professionals verify the compound's contents. It also meets USP and state regulations for compounded product labeling and promotes patient safety.

Q313. Answer: B

Explanation: When a patient requests a generic substitution, the technician must confirm substitution is permitted by state law and the prescription itself, then notify the pharmacist. Only the pharmacist can authorize substitution after verifying equivalency. This process ensures therapeutic consistency, cost-effectiveness, and compliance with legal substitution guidelines while maintaining patient trust and safety.

Q314. Answer: A

Explanation: Before processing a refill request, the technician must check the prescription number and the number of remaining authorized refills. This verification prevents unauthorized refills and ensures legal compliance. It also confirms that the patient continues therapy safely under prescriber approval, maintaining accurate recordkeeping and continuity of care in the pharmacy workflow.

Q315. Answer: B

Explanation: A verbal prescription must include the prescriber's name and DEA number if it involves controlled substances. These details verify the prescriber's authority and ensure the prescription's legality. The technician's responsibility is to transcribe the order accurately and confirm all essential elements before pharmacist review, ensuring compliance and safe medication dispensing.

Q316. Answer: C

Explanation: If a drug interaction alert appears, the technician must immediately notify the pharmacist. Only the pharmacist can assess the clinical significance and determine whether to proceed. Technicians play a vital safety role by identifying and escalating potential issues, ensuring no harmful combinations are dispensed and maintaining high standards of patient safety and legal compliance.

Q317. Answer: B

Explanation: Recording lot numbers ensures traceability of ingredients in case of a recall or adverse event. This documentation allows the pharmacy to identify affected products quickly, protecting patient safety and maintaining compliance with USP and FDA standards. It provides an audit trail essential for quality control and accountability in pharmacy operations.

Q318. Answer: B

Explanation: Rotating inventory so older stock is used first (first-expired, first-out method) prevents medication waste and ensures drugs are dispensed while still effective. This practice supports efficient inventory control, minimizes losses, and maintains product integrity. Proper stock rotation ensures patients receive medications with valid expiration dates, enhancing both safety and cost efficiency.

Q319. Answer: A

Explanation: Before compounding an IV admixture, technicians must verify all ingredients and check for compatibility. Incompatibilities can cause precipitation or loss of potency, risking patient safety. This verification ensures proper formulation, accurate concentrations, and adherence to USP <797> standards for sterile compounding, ensuring that the product is safe and effective for patient use.

Q320. Answer: B

Explanation: Controlled substances require documentation of the prescriber's DEA number and a complete dispensing record. This ensures traceability, prevents diversion, and supports DEA audits. Technicians help maintain these records accurately for legal compliance and accountability. Proper documentation ensures that controlled substances are dispensed safely and in accordance with strict federal regulations.

Q321. Answer: B

Explanation: Verifying the correct concentration and providing an appropriate measuring device ensures dosing accuracy for liquid medications. Incorrect concentrations or missing devices can cause serious underdosing or overdosing. Technicians play a critical role in checking liquid formulations to maintain accuracy, promote proper patient use, and prevent medication administration errors.

Q322. Answer: A

Explanation: The technician must ensure that the directions on the printed label exactly match the prescriber's original instructions. Consistency between the prescription and label ensures safe and accurate medication use. Any discrepancies can lead to dosing errors or misunderstandings. This accuracy is a fundamental responsibility in the prescription filling process.

Q323. Answer: B

Explanation: Each unit-dose package must display the drug name, strength, and expiration date. This labeling ensures correct identification and prevents medication errors during administration. It also complies with FDA and USP guidelines for repackaged drug labeling, maintaining patient safety and facilitating efficient verification by healthcare providers during medication administration.

Q324. Answer: D

Explanation: The laminar airflow hood must be cleaned before each sterile compounding session, after spills, and periodically during extended use. This prevents contamination and ensures aseptic conditions. Regular cleaning with approved disinfectants maintains sterility, complies with USP <797> standards, and protects patients from potential microbial contamination in compounded sterile products.

Q325. Answer: B

Explanation: If a technician observes a foreign particle in a sterile preparation, the solution must be discarded immediately and reported to the pharmacist. Contamination compromises product sterility and patient safety. Discarding ensures no contaminated medication is dispensed, maintaining compliance with USP <797> and sterile compounding safety standards.

Q326. Answer: B

Explanation: Proper hand hygiene involves washing hands and forearms thoroughly with soap and water for at least 30 seconds before compounding. This removes microorganisms and prevents contamination of sterile products. This practice complies with USP <797> standards and ensures aseptic technique integrity, protecting patients from infection and ensuring product sterility.

Q327. Answer: A

Explanation: Documenting a compounding error immediately promotes transparency, helps identify root causes, and supports corrective action to prevent recurrence. Reporting errors ensures accountability, continuous quality improvement, and patient safety. It also fulfills regulatory obligations for incident documentation and helps maintain trust and integrity within the pharmacy practice environment.

Q328. Answer: A

Explanation: Before counting, the technician must verify that the manufacturer's bottle NDC, drug name, and strength match the prescription label. This ensures accurate drug selection and prevents mix-ups between similar products. Verification protects patient safety, ensures consistency, and supports pharmacist validation prior to dispensing, maintaining regulatory and safety standards.

Q329. Answer: B

Explanation: Bar-code verification systems ensure that the correct drug is matched with the correct patient and prescription. Scanning reduces human error by verifying product information electronically before dispensing. This system strengthens medication safety, supports inventory accuracy, and improves workflow efficiency while maintaining compliance with pharmacy technology best practices.

Q330. Answer: A

Explanation: Double-count verification should be performed for all medications, with special emphasis on controlled substances. This ensures that the dispensed quantity matches the prescription exactly and prevents significant errors. It also maintains compliance with controlled substance regulations, ensuring accountability and accuracy throughout the dispensing process.

Q331. Answer: B

Explanation: The date of dispensing must be included on every prescription label to document when the medication was prepared and released. This information aids in recordkeeping, helps track expiration timelines, and ensures regulatory compliance. It also assists in verifying when refills or follow-up prescriptions may be due, ensuring proper medication management.

Q332. Answer: A

Explanation: Maintaining sterility requires preventing contact between sterile and non-sterile surfaces. This protects compounded products from contamination during transfers and manipulations. Technicians must work within the airflow hood and handle materials correctly to preserve aseptic conditions, ensuring compliance with USP <797> and the safety of sterile preparations for patient use.

Q333. Answer: C

Explanation: Each compounded batch must include detailed records of the technician's name, ingredient lot numbers, and exact quantities used. These records ensure traceability, quality control, and accountability. Accurate documentation supports audits, facilitates recalls if needed, and ensures the compounded product meets regulatory and safety standards set by USP and FDA.

Q334. Answer: A

Explanation: Antibiotic suspensions must be reconstituted with the exact amount of diluent specified by the manufacturer before dispensing. Proper reconstitution ensures correct concentration and therapeutic effect. Technicians must measure accurately and shake the mixture to uniformity, ensuring the product is safe, effective, and ready for immediate use upon pharmacist verification.

Q335. Answer: A

Explanation: Storage instructions guide patients and healthcare providers on maintaining medication stability and potency. Proper storage prevents degradation, contamination, or loss of efficacy. By including clear storage directions, technicians ensure the medication remains effective until its expiration, promoting patient safety and compliance with regulatory labeling requirements.

Q336. Answer: A

Explanation: Before printing a label, the technician must ensure that all entered data—patient name, drug name, strength, dosage, and directions—matches the original prescription exactly. Label accuracy ensures the correct medication is dispensed and used safely by the patient. This verification prevents errors, supports pharmacist review, and fulfills legal labeling and safety standards.

Q337. Answer: B

Explanation: Expired controlled substances must be segregated and documented for pharmacist review before proper disposal. The pharmacist oversees return or destruction according to DEA Form 41 regulations. Technicians ensure accurate documentation and secure handling to prevent diversion, maintain legal compliance, and protect patient safety by ensuring expired medications are never dispensed.

Q338. Answer: B

Explanation: Schedule III–V controlled substances may be transferred once between pharmacies for refill purposes, provided DEA and state rules are followed. The technician assists by accurately recording transfer details and verifying authorization. This process ensures accountability, legal compliance, and prevents duplicate dispensing or diversion of controlled medications.

Q339. Answer: A

Explanation: Recording expiration dates on repackaged items ensures that medications are used before they expire and that no expired products are dispensed. This maintains product potency, protects patient health, and supports compliance with USP and FDA labeling standards. Proper expiration tracking also facilitates safe stock rotation and quality control in pharmacy operations.

Q340. Answer: D

Explanation: During the pharmacist's final check, the technician's role is to ensure that labeling, packaging, and prescription information are error-free before presentation. This step ensures a smooth verification process. Although the pharmacist performs the clinical review, the technician's attention to detail supports safety, efficiency, and accuracy during the final verification.

Q341. Answer: A

Explanation: Returning controlled substances to the supplier requires completing DEA Form 222, which authorizes and documents the transaction. This ensures legal accountability and traceability of controlled medications. Technicians assist by maintaining accurate inventory records and securing products until the return is processed. Proper documentation prevents diversion and ensures compliance with DEA regulations.

Q342. Answer: A

Explanation: Maintaining patient confidentiality is a core responsibility. Technicians must discuss prescription details only with the patient, prescriber, or pharmacist. This protects patient privacy under HIPAA regulations, prevents unauthorized disclosure of sensitive information, and builds trust between the patient and pharmacy. Confidential handling safeguards both ethical and legal pharmacy standards.

Q343. Answer: B

Explanation: Every prescription label must contain the patient's name, the drug name, and clear dosage directions. These details ensure that patients can correctly identify and use their medications as prescribed. Accurate labeling supports safe administration, prevents confusion, and meets state and federal labeling requirements essential for effective pharmacy practice.

Q344. Answer: A

Explanation: Disinfecting vial stoppers with 70% isopropyl alcohol before puncture prevents contamination of sterile solutions. This step is critical in aseptic compounding to maintain sterility within the laminar airflow hood. Following USP <797> procedures ensures patient safety by preventing microbial introduction into compounded sterile preparations.

Q345. Answer: B

Explanation: A unit-dose package must display the drug name, strength, lot number, and expiration date. These elements provide traceability, ensure proper identification, and allow verification before administration. Accurate labeling prevents medication errors in healthcare settings and complies with USP and FDA requirements for unit-dose systems.

Q346. Answer: A

Explanation: Using a clean counting tray and spatula for each medication prevents cross-contamination and ensures accuracy. Residue from previous drugs can cause allergic reactions or dosing errors. Proper hygiene and counting practices uphold quality control, maintain patient safety, and align with pharmacy operational standards.

Q347. Answer: A

Explanation: Antineoplastic drugs must always be handled in a biological safety cabinet due to their hazardous and carcinogenic properties. This containment prevents technician exposure and environmental contamination. Following USP <800> and OSHA guidelines ensures safety, compliance, and protection of pharmacy personnel handling these high-risk medications.

Q348. Answer: D

Explanation: When a third-party claim is rejected, the technician reviews the reason, attempts to resolve the billing issue, and alerts the pharmacist. This ensures the patient can access medication promptly without unnecessary delays. Accurate handling of insurance rejections maintains efficiency and compliance with insurance and pharmacy protocols.

Q349. Answer: B

Explanation: When a balance due notice appears, the technician should inform the patient courteously and attempt to reprocess the claim if possible. Effective communication maintains trust and ensures accurate billing. Handling financial alerts properly supports workflow efficiency while adhering to insurance and payment protocols without compromising patient service.

Q350. Answer: A

Explanation: Repackaged bulk medications must carry a new label containing the drug name, strength, lot number, and beyond-use date. This labeling ensures traceability, stability, and patient safety. Technicians maintain documentation for quality control and compliance with USP <795> and FDA regulations for repackaged pharmaceutical products.

Q351. Answer: A

Explanation: Upon receiving a recall alert, the technician must isolate the affected medication to prevent further dispensing. This prevents patients from receiving potentially unsafe products. After isolation, the pharmacist reviews and determines next steps for returning or disposing of the product according to recall instructions, ensuring safety and compliance.

Q352. Answer: A

Explanation: DEA Form 106 is used to report the loss or theft of controlled substances. This mandatory report ensures accountability and compliance with DEA regulations. Technicians assist by documenting inventory discrepancies and providing details for the report. Prompt submission protects against diversion and maintains regulatory integrity within pharmacy operations.

Q353. Answer: C

Explanation: If a forged or suspicious prescription is identified, the technician must alert the pharmacist immediately. The pharmacist will verify authenticity and, if necessary, contact law enforcement or the prescriber. This prevents illegal dispensing, protects the pharmacy's license, and maintains compliance with DEA and state laws.

Q354. Answer: A

Explanation: Label reconciliation involves confirming that the printed label matches the prescription and selected product precisely. This step ensures medication accuracy, proper instructions, and patient safety. Technicians play a vital role by verifying all printed information before the pharmacist's final check, minimizing labeling errors and ensuring accurate dispensing.

Q355. Answer: A

Explanation: Hazardous waste from compounding must be disposed of according to OSHA and EPA regulations using labeled, sealed containers. This prevents environmental contamination and technician exposure. Compliance ensures workplace safety and adherence to USP <800> requirements for hazardous drug management in the pharmacy setting.

Q356. Answer: C

Explanation: When a prescriber cancels a prescription, the technician must mark it as "void" and record the cancellation in the patient's profile. This maintains accurate records, prevents accidental dispensing, and complies with pharmacy documentation standards. Proper cancellation tracking also supports legal accountability and patient safety.

Q357. Answer: A

Explanation: During controlled substance inventory, the technician must count and document quantities accurately to ensure compliance with DEA requirements. This helps detect discrepancies, prevents diversion, and maintains an accurate record of stock. Thorough and precise counting supports accountability and ensures the pharmacy meets legal inventory standards.

Q358. Answer: A

Explanation: Auxiliary labels provide essential warnings such as "May cause drowsiness" or "Avoid sunlight," guiding safe medication use. Proper application ensures patients are informed of precautions that can prevent adverse effects or misuse. These labels complement pharmacist counseling and reinforce patient understanding, promoting safe and effective therapy.

Q359. Answer: B

Explanation: Technicians maintain automated dispensing systems by verifying calibration, cleanliness, and correct medication loading. These tasks prevent dispensing errors and ensure system accuracy. Routine maintenance also includes checking expiration dates and clearing alerts. Proper upkeep ensures reliability and compliance with safety protocols in automated medication distribution.

Q360. Answer: A

Explanation: Matching the label to the stock bottle confirms the correct medication and strength were used in filling. This final verification before pharmacist review prevents dispensing errors. Technicians ensure label and product consistency to maintain accuracy, safety, and compliance with pharmacy verification procedures, ultimately protecting patient well-being.

Q361. Answer: D

Explanation: Before filling a prescription, verifying patient identity and prescription validity ensures accuracy and legal compliance. Confirming this information prevents errors caused by duplicate names or fraudulent prescriptions. This step guarantees that the correct medication is being prepared for the right patient under valid authorization, forming the foundation for safe and efficient dispensing.

Q362. Answer: A

Explanation: A perpetual inventory maintains real-time records of all controlled substance transactions, enabling immediate identification of discrepancies or diversion. Continuous monitoring promotes accountability, supports DEA compliance, and protects public safety. Technicians assist in updating this record with each transaction, ensuring precise tracking of controlled drugs from receipt to dispensing.

Q363. Answer: A

Explanation: Cytotoxic medications must be handled using full protective gear (gloves, gown, mask) and inside a biological safety cabinet. These drugs pose carcinogenic and mutagenic risks if mishandled. Following USP <800> and OSHA standards minimizes exposure and contamination, protecting both pharmacy staff and the environment from hazardous drug particles or vapors.

Q364. Answer: D

Explanation: The technician must verify that the medication and quantity in the container match the prescription before labeling. Applying a label prematurely could result in labeling errors or incorrect drug dispensation. Confirming these details ensures alignment with the prescriber's order, enhances safety, and maintains workflow accuracy during the pharmacist's final verification.

Q365. Answer: A

Explanation: Upon identifying a duplicate prescription, the technician must alert the pharmacist immediately. Duplicate prescriptions can lead to double dosing or misuse if processed incorrectly. The pharmacist will verify the intent with the prescriber before deciding how to proceed. Early recognition by the technician prevents potential medication errors and ensures compliance.

Q366. Answer: A

Explanation: REMS programs are required for medications with serious safety concerns. They include specific dispensing, monitoring, and counseling steps to protect patients. Technicians help ensure all REMS criteria—such as authorization codes or enrollment forms—are met before dispensing. These safeguards prevent inappropriate medication use and adverse outcomes, maintaining compliance with FDA safety protocols.

Q367. Answer: B

Explanation: Processing one prescription at a time ensures accuracy and minimizes errors caused by distractions during busy periods. Sequential workflow helps technicians maintain focus, prevents mix-ups, and supports accurate verification of each prescription component. This method promotes consistent safety and reliability within high-volume pharmacy environments.

Q368. Answer: A

Explanation: Preventing contamination during sterile compounding requires adherence to aseptic technique and use of sterile, disinfected equipment. This includes proper garbing, handwashing, and working in a certified laminar airflow hood. Compliance with USP <797> ensures sterility, reduces infection risk, and guarantees patient safety through contamination-free compounded preparations.

Q369. Answer: C

Explanation: Accurate patient profiles contain essential information such as allergies, current medications, and medical history. Keeping these updated helps the pharmacist identify potential interactions or duplicate therapies before dispensing. This record ensures continuity of care, supports medication safety, and complies with pharmacy documentation standards for patient protection.

Q370. Answer: A

Explanation: Most reconstituted antibiotic suspensions must be refrigerated at 2–8°C to maintain stability and potency until the beyond-use date. Proper storage prevents bacterial degradation and ensures effectiveness throughout the treatment period. Technicians must verify manufacturer instructions to ensure the correct temperature for each specific formulation.

Q371. Answer: A

Explanation: Calibration ensures that measuring devices deliver precise quantities of ingredients, which is critical for accuracy in compounded preparations. Proper calibration maintains consistency, prevents dosing errors, and ensures that compounded medications meet quality and potency standards required under USP <795> and <797> regulations.

Q372. Answer: A

Explanation: Federal labeling requirements mandate that directions for use and the prescriber's name appear on every prescription label. This ensures clarity and accountability, allowing patients to follow correct dosing schedules and identify who prescribed the medication. It supports safe use, effective therapy, and compliance with labeling laws.

Q373. Answer: B

Explanation: Verifying the DEA number ensures that the prescriber is authorized to prescribe controlled substances. The technician checks validity by performing a simple calculation where the final digit matches the check digit. This verification prevents fraudulent prescriptions and ensures compliance with DEA and state controlled substance laws.

Q374. Answer: A

Explanation: Verifying the patient's identifying information ensures that the correct profile is created and prevents future mix-ups or misfiled prescriptions. Accurate data entry allows proper tracking of medication history, insurance coverage, and allergy information. This step ensures continuity of care and compliance with patient verification protocols.

Q375. Answer: C

Explanation: A complete compounding record includes ingredients used, their quantities, lot numbers, and the assigned beyond-use date. This documentation ensures traceability, reproducibility, and accountability. It allows verification of accuracy and quality control for each compounded preparation, supporting USP and FDA compliance while ensuring patient safety.

Q376. Answer: A

Explanation: If a prescription SIG (directions for use) is unclear, the technician must notify the pharmacist immediately. Only the pharmacist can clarify instructions with the prescriber. This prevents misinterpretation and ensures that the patient receives the correct dosage and usage information, maintaining safety and compliance with prescription accuracy standards.

Q377. Answer: A

Explanation: Light-sensitive medications must be stored in amber or opaque containers to protect against light degradation, which can reduce potency and effectiveness. This precaution ensures drug stability and extends shelf life. Technicians must follow manufacturer and USP recommendations for light protection to preserve medication quality and efficacy.

Q378. Answer: D

Explanation: Documenting refrigerator temperatures ensures that medications requiring cold storage are maintained within safe, effective ranges (typically 2–8°C). Consistent monitoring prevents loss of potency or spoilage. Technicians log readings regularly to verify compliance with USP, FDA, and manufacturer storage standards, ensuring product integrity and patient safety.

Q379. Answer: A

Explanation: Before returning a medication bottle to stock, the technician must verify that it remains sealed, untampered, and unexpired. This ensures product safety and prevents dispensing compromised medications. Proper inspection maintains inventory integrity, patient trust, and compliance with storage and dispensing regulations.

Q380. Answer: A

Explanation: Uniform, homogeneous mixing ensures that active ingredients are evenly distributed in topical ointments, providing consistent therapeutic effect with each dose. This precision prevents over- or underdosing in localized areas. Following compounding procedures guarantees product quality, stability, and compliance with USP <795> standards for non-sterile preparations.

Q381. Answer: B

Explanation: Accurate entry of prescription and patient data before claim submission ensures correct insurance billing and prevents rejections. This includes entering the correct NDC, quantity, and patient identifiers. Precise data management supports smooth reimbursement, reduces claim errors, and maintains compliance with third-party billing requirements.

Q382. Answer: A

Explanation: Controlled substances require double verification of every transaction and proper signature logs to ensure accountability and traceability. This prevents diversion and maintains compliance with DEA regulations. Having two staff members verify and sign off adds an essential safeguard against discrepancies and ensures secure management of controlled inventory.

Q383. Answer: D

Explanation: Frequent cleaning of pharmacy work surfaces prevents contamination, supports aseptic technique, and maintains the integrity of prepared medications. Cleaning removes residue, dust, and potential cross-contaminants that could affect product safety. This practice aligns with USP and OSHA standards, ensuring a hygienic environment for compounding and dispensing operations.

Q384. Answer: A

Explanation: Verifying the device type, dose counter, and correct labeling ensures the patient receives the correct inhaler form and dose. This prevents confusion between different inhalers with similar names but varying functions. Proper verification supports patient adherence, medication safety, and accurate use instructions under pharmacist supervision.

Q385. Answer: A

Explanation: Before dispensing reconstituted ophthalmic solutions, the technician must ensure sterility, correct dilution, and accurate beyond-use dating. These checks prevent infection risk and guarantee potency throughout the medication's use. Proper handling of reconstituted eye drops ensures compliance with USP <797> sterile compounding standards and patient safety in ophthalmic therapy.

Q386. Answer: C

Explanation: Recording the lot number allows traceability in case of recalls, contamination, or reported adverse effects. This information identifies the exact product batch dispensed, ensuring patient safety and regulatory compliance. It supports quality control, facilitates prompt recall responses, and aligns with FDA and pharmacy documentation standards for accountability and tracking purposes.

Q387. Answer: A

Explanation: The technician ensures that the prescription is completely filled, correctly labeled, and ready for pharmacist review. This includes verifying medication strength, dosage form, and quantity. Proper preparation minimizes pharmacist corrections, enhances efficiency, and supports patient safety by allowing the pharmacist to focus solely on clinical verification and final approval.

Q388. Answer: B

Explanation: Before compounding an IV admixture, technicians must verify that all ingredients are compatible and that the correct diluent is used. This ensures the stability and safety of the final product. Incompatible ingredients can precipitate, degrade, or harm the patient. Verifying compatibility is crucial for compliance with USP <797> standards and aseptic integrity.

Q389. Answer: A

Explanation: Storing high-alert medications separately helps prevent selection or dispensing errors that could cause significant patient harm. Isolating drugs like insulin or anticoagulants ensures extra caution during handling and verification. This practice aligns with ISMP safety recommendations, enhances workflow awareness, and promotes safer pharmacy operations through physical and procedural safeguards.

Q390. Answer: A

Explanation: Early refill requests for controlled substances require immediate pharmacist attention. The pharmacist verifies refill eligibility with the prescriber and ensures compliance with DEA regulations. Technicians must not approve such requests independently, as unauthorized dispensing may violate laws and increase diversion risk. Prompt communication preserves compliance and ensures patient safety.

Q391. Answer: C

Explanation: Clear, legible labels ensure that patients can easily understand dosage instructions and warnings, reducing the risk of misuse or nonadherence. Label clarity enhances safety, supports literacy needs, and complies with FDA and state regulations requiring legible prescription instructions. It is vital for proper medication administration and patient trust.

Q392. Answer: A

Explanation: The technician must add the precise amount of diluent specified by the manufacturer to ensure correct concentration and stability. Deviating from this amount can alter dosing accuracy and therapeutic effectiveness. Using purified or distilled water and following manufacturer directions guarantee uniformity, potency, and patient safety in reconstituted oral medications.

Q393. Answer: D

Explanation: When transferring a prescription, the technician must document complete transfer details, including the original and receiving pharmacy names, prescription number, and date of transfer. This ensures continuity of care, prevents duplicate dispensing, and complies with state and DEA recordkeeping laws. Accurate documentation protects patient safety and maintains legal accountability.

Q394. Answer: A

Explanation: Beyond-use dating defines the time frame within which a medication remains stable and effective after preparation or reconstitution. This ensures patients receive products that maintain potency and safety. Assigning accurate BUDs per USP <795> or <797> standards prevents degradation-related errors and guarantees the quality of compounded or reconstituted medications.

Q395. Answer: A

Explanation: Verifying the drug name, strength, and NDC ensures the correct medication is selected from inventory. The NDC uniquely identifies the manufacturer and product formulation, helping prevent mix-ups with look-alike or sound-alike drugs. This verification is a critical accuracy checkpoint that supports safe dispensing and compliance with pharmacy standards.

Q396. Answer: B

Explanation: Using a clean, designated counting tray and verifying totals before labeling ensures correct quantities and prevents cross-contamination. Accurate counting is essential for safe dosing, particularly for controlled or narrow-therapeutic-index drugs. Double-checking counts enhances accuracy, accountability, and compliance with pharmacy quality assurance practices.

Q397. Answer: A

Explanation: Confirming prescriber credentials ensures that the individual is authorized to prescribe the specific medication, particularly controlled substances. This verification prevents fraudulent or invalid prescriptions, maintains legal compliance, and safeguards patient safety. Technicians assist by verifying DEA numbers and state licensure, ensuring all prescriptions meet regulatory authorization standards.

Q398. Answer: A

Explanation: Reviewing prescriptions for completeness and legibility prevents data entry errors and ensures all required details—such as patient name, medication, dosage, and prescriber—are accurate. Identifying missing or unclear information early allows correction before processing, avoiding potential dispensing errors and promoting efficiency and safety in pharmacy workflow.

Q399. Answer: C

Explanation: Before dispensing, technicians must verify that sterile products are clear, free of particulates, and labeled correctly. Visual inspection ensures integrity and sterility compliance under USP <797>. Detecting abnormalities early prevents unsafe administration, ensuring patient protection and adherence to sterile preparation quality standards.

Q400. Answer: A

Explanation: Hazardous drugs must be compounded within a biological safety cabinet (BSC) or compounding aseptic containment isolator (CACI) to prevent exposure and environmental contamination. These engineering controls protect technicians and maintain negative pressure environments. Following USP <800> ensures safety, compliance, and containment during hazardous drug preparation.

Questions (401-500)

Q401. What information must appear on all compounded product labels?

A. Name, strength, beyond-use date, and storage instructions
B. Patient's insurance ID
C. Pharmacy website address
D. Manufacturer's advertising tagline

Q402. What step prevents cross-contamination when compounding?

A. Mixing multiple drugs at once
B. Using the same mortar and pestle for all drugs
C. Cleaning equipment and workspace before and after each use
D. Skipping garbing procedures

Q403. Why must beyond-use dates (BUDs) be applied to compounded products?

A. To indicate how long the compound remains stable and effective
B. To identify when it was ordered
C. To match billing cycles
D. To comply with brand labeling

Q404. What is required for proper documentation of sterile compounding?

A. Record of ingredients, lot numbers, quantities, and preparation date
B. Pharmacist's favorite brand
C. Patient's insurance code
D. Supplier's contact list

Q405建议. Why should technicians perform double verification on controlled medications?

A. To simplify recordkeeping
B. To expedite workflow
C. To reduce pharmacist involvement
D. To ensure accuracy, accountability, and DEA compliance

Q406. Which of the following is a technician's duty during refill authorization requests?

A. Forwarding refill requests to the prescriber for approval
B. Approving refills independently
C. Changing directions based on patient request
D. Issuing extra medication for convenience

Q407. Why must hazardous drug waste be disposed of in designated containers?

A. To prevent exposure, contamination, and environmental harm
B. To save space in regular waste bins
C. To meet customer service goals
D. To reduce recycling costs

Q408. What must a technician confirm before labeling repackaged unit doses?

A. Only patient initials
B. Correct drug name, strength, lot number, and expiration date
C. Prescription price
D. Drug color

Q409. Why must all measuring devices used for liquids be specific to the medication?

A. To ensure precise dosing accuracy for each formulation
B. To simplify inventory
C. To reduce waste
D. To avoid patient questions

Q410. When compounding non-sterile preparations, why must ingredient weights be verified twice?

A. To avoid excess paperwork
B. To record the technician's speed
C. To ensure formulation accuracy and product consistency
D. To simplify cleanup

Q411. Why must compounded products be labeled with storage instructions?
A. To ensure stability and prevent degradation under improper conditions
B. To advertise the pharmacy's name
C. To meet insurance documentation requirements
D. To remind patients of dosage timing

Q412. Before compounding a sterile product, what should the technician confirm about all vials and containers?
A. Integrity of seals, expiration dates, and particulate-free solutions
B. Manufacturer's sales record
C. Patient's billing details
D. Pharmacist's shift time

Q413. Which procedure ensures proper drug identification before counting tablets?
A. Matching manufacturer location
B. Checking bottle color only
C. Relying on memory of packaging
D. Comparing NDC number, drug name, and strength with the prescription

Q414. When preparing sterile IV medications, what is the primary aseptic goal?
A. Preventing microbial contamination of compounded products
B. Reducing inventory waste
C. Increasing preparation speed
D. Improving product color

Q415. What is the technician's first responsibility when identifying a prescription error?
A. Stop processing and inform the pharmacist immediately
B. Correct it independently
C. Notify the patient directly
D. Continue processing to save time

Q416. Which medication should always be kept in its original packaging due to sensitivity?
A. Ibuprofen tablets
B. Amoxicillin capsules
C. Nitroglycerin sublingual tablets
D. Loratadine chewables

Q417. Why is recordkeeping crucial for all compounded medications?
A. It ensures traceability, accountability, and regulatory compliance
B. It serves as advertising for the pharmacy
C. It increases workflow efficiency
D. It replaces pharmacist verification

Q418. What must a technician verify when a prescription contains multiple strengths of the same drug?
A. Select the higher strength automatically
B. Confirm the prescribed strength matches the SIG and prescriber's intent
C. Dispense both strengths together
D. Ask the patient to decide

Q419. Which task ensures compliance with DEA regulations for controlled substances?
A. Maintaining complete and accurate dispensing logs
B. Using generic substitutions

C. Allowing early refills
D. Storing them with OTC medications
Q420. What is required before a technician can fill a new prescription for a patient?
A. Verification of patient allergies and demographic information
B. Only the patient's phone number
C. Pharmacist's initials
D. The patient's insurance card
Q421. Why should look-alike/sound-alike drugs be stored separately?
A. To make inventory audits easier
B. To increase visual appeal of shelving
C. To speed up dispensing
D. To prevent selection and dispensing errors due to confusion
Q422. What must be verified before labeling a controlled medication?
A. DEA number and number of authorized refills
B. Patient's nickname
C. Pharmacy manager's credentials
D. Manufacturer's logo
Q423. What is the purpose of a sterile media fill test in compounding?
A. To verify prescription entry accuracy
B. To assess aseptic technique and contamination prevention skills
C. To test drug potency
D. To evaluate inventory control
Q424. Why should single-use vials not be reused once opened?
A. They lack preservatives and risk contamination
B. They are too costly to reuse
C. They cause dosage inconsistencies
D. They expire only after 30 days
Q425. When processing a faxed prescription, the technician must first:
A. Confirm authenticity and prescriber information before entry
B. Enter it without review
C. Call the patient for confirmation
D. File it immediately
Q426. Which key step prevents transcription errors during prescription data entry?
A. Skipping patient verification
B. Entering data without review
C. Reading back and confirming the entered data
D. Using abbreviations inconsistently
Q427. Why should hazardous drug spill kits be accessible in the pharmacy?
A. To safely contain and clean accidental hazardous material spills
B. To store extra gloves
C. To speed up workflow
D. To manage temperature control
Q428. What is the technician's duty regarding expired medications on the shelf?
A. Remove them promptly and document for disposal
B. Dispense them if color appears normal
C. Hide them behind new stock
D. Use them for compounding
Q429. When handling a temperature excursion alert for refrigerated drugs, the technician should:

A. Reset the refrigerator
B. Ignore it if the power returns quickly
C. Continue dispensing
D. Quarantine affected items and notify the pharmacist

Q430. Why should compounded sterile preparations (CSPs) be visually inspected before release?
A. To detect particulates, discoloration, or container defects
B. To confirm label design
C. To evaluate cost-effectiveness
D. To ensure storage space efficiency

Q431. Which piece of information is mandatory on controlled substance prescription labels?
A. Patient's nickname
B. Federal transfer warning statement
C. Insurance plan type
D. Technician initials

Q432. What must a technician verify before labeling a compounded topical cream?
A. Ingredient accuracy, concentration, and beyond-use date
B. Manufacturer's phone number
C. Cream texture and color preference
D. Patient's copay

Q433. Why are independent double checks important for high-risk preparations?
A. They confirm accuracy of critical steps and reduce error risk
B. They delay workflow for redundancy
C. They replace pharmacist verification
D. They ensure faster documentation

Q434. What should a technician do if foreign particles are seen in a sterile vial?
A. Shake it to dissolve
B. Use it after filtering
C. Discard the vial immediately and notify the pharmacist
D. Label it for future use

Q435. Why must airflow hoods be certified regularly in sterile compounding areas?
A. To ensure they provide proper laminar airflow and sterility protection
B. To reduce pharmacy noise
C. To increase storage capacity
D. To meet aesthetic standards

Q436. (Prescription Intake) When a new patient presents a prescription, what must be verified before processing?
A. Patient identity and date of birth
B. Prescription color
C. Drug manufacturer name
D. Insurance group number

Q437. (Dispensing) What is the correct step when a medication stock bottle's label is unreadable?
A. Continue dispensing to avoid delay
B. Use it if the NDC seems familiar
C. Replace the label yourself
D. Quarantine the bottle and notify the pharmacist

Q438. (Calculations) How many milliliters are needed to provide a 10-day supply if the patient takes 10 mL three times daily?
A. 300 mL

B. 150 mL
C. 100 mL
D. 200 mL

Q439. (Compounding) What is the correct sequence before compounding a sterile product?

A. Prepare ingredients first
B. Perform hand hygiene, garbing, and surface disinfection
C. Adjust laminar hood airflow
D. Label vials before cleaning

Q440. (Intake) What should a technician do if a prescription has illegible directions?

A. Hold it and ask the pharmacist to clarify with the prescriber
B. Interpret it personally
C. Fill it as written
D. Ask the patient to guess

Q441. (Dispensing) Why must auxiliary labels be applied when indicated?

A. To make containers uniform
B. To decorate prescription bottles
C. To meet inventory audits
D. To communicate critical usage or safety information to patients

Q442. (Calculations) Convert 2 grams of medication to milligrams.

A. 2000 mg
B. 20 mg
C. 0.2 mg
D. 200 mg

Q443. (Compounding) Why should beyond-use dates be assigned to all compounded preparations?

A. To specify how long the product remains safe and effective
B. To determine the pharmacist's schedule
C. To calculate profit margin
D. To match packaging dates

Q444. (Intake) What should a technician confirm before entering insurance information?

A. That the patient's name and date of birth match the insurance card
B. That coverage includes brand drugs
C. That the insurer is local
D. That the pharmacist has approved it

Q445. (Dispensing) Why must controlled substances be double-counted before dispensing?

A. To reduce pharmacist workload
B. To confirm label alignment
C. To verify accuracy and prevent diversion
D. To track refill dates

Q446. (Calculations) A prescription reads: "Amoxicillin 250 mg/5 mL, 1 teaspoon TID for 10 days." How many mL are needed?

A. 150 mL
B. 100 mL
C. 200 mL
D. 250 mL

Q447. (Compounding) Why are calibrated devices used in compounding?

A. To measure ingredients accurately and ensure formulation precision
B. To speed up production
C. To avoid pharmacist supervision

D. To meet marketing requirements

Q448. (Intake) Which action ensures HIPAA compliance during prescription processing?

A. Confirming details loudly at the counter

B. Discussing patient details privately

C. Leaving profiles open on shared screens

D. Sharing data with insurance marketers

Q449. (Dispensing) Why must medications with look-alike packaging be stored separately?

A. To reduce the risk of selection and dispensing errors

B. To enhance storage aesthetics

C. To increase shelving capacity

D. To simplify barcode scanning

Q450. (Calculations) If 120 mL of solution contains 480 mg of drug, how many mg are in 30 mL?

A. 120 mg

B. 480 mg

C. 240 mg

D. 60 mg

Q451. (Compounding) Why must compounded sterile products be visually inspected before release?

A. To check for particulate matter, clarity, and color consistency

B. To verify packaging style

C. To confirm insurance status

D. To match label colors

Q452. (Intake) What documentation is required when transferring a prescription between pharmacies?

A. Manufacturer's ID code

B. Patient's social security number

C. Insurance premiums

D. Prescription number, dates, and pharmacy identifiers

Q453. (Dispensing) Why must expiration dates be checked before filling prescriptions?

A. To ensure medication potency and safety

B. To match packaging lots

C. To assist marketing analysis

D. To calculate pricing

Q454. (Calculations) A 2% w/v solution means how many grams of solute in 100 mL?

A. 2 g

B. 20 g

C. 0.2 g

D. 10 g

Q455. (Compounding) Why must non-sterile compounding areas be kept clean and organized?

A. To reduce packaging costs

B. To improve pharmacy appearance

C. To prevent cross-contamination and maintain product integrity

D. To pass marketing inspections

Q456. (Intake) What must a technician confirm before entering a verbal prescription?

A. Accurate spelling, dosage, and prescriber details

B. Patient's insurance price

C. Preferred pharmacy color scheme

D. Manufacturer rebate

Q457. (Dispensing) What is the purpose of unit-dose packaging in institutional settings?

A. To ensure accurate administration and reduce medication errors

B. To simplify billing
C. To promote manufacturer sales
D. To reduce inventory counts

Q458. (Calculations) How many milligrams are in 250 mL of a 4 mg/mL solution?
A. 1000 mg
B. 500 mg
C. 1500 mg
D. 200 mg

Q459. (Compounding) Why must all equipment used in compounding be properly cleaned and dried before use?
A. To speed production
B. To prevent contamination and ensure ingredient accuracy
C. To reduce calibration needs
D. To increase shelf life

Q460. (Intake) Why must technicians check for drug interactions during order entry?
A. To assist the pharmacist in identifying potential conflicts before dispensing
B. To expedite billing
C. To increase prescription volume
D. To substitute generics independently

Q461. Before processing any prescription, what must the technician confirm about the prescriber's order?
A. Drug manufacturer preference
B. Patient's payment history
C. Completeness, legibility, and authenticity
D. Insurance billing codes

Q462. Why is it essential to verify that a prescription quantity and SIG match logically?
A. To ensure the medication can be used as prescribed for the intended duration
B. To simplify label printing
C. To adjust inventory counts
D. To speed up processing

Q463. A patient is prescribed 500 mg tablets, two tablets every 8 hours for 10 days. How many tablets are needed?
A. 40
B. 60
C. 20
D. 30

Q464. Why must a technician verify that a medication bottle's barcode matches the prescription?
A. To ensure correct product selection and reduce dispensing errors
B. To confirm packaging aesthetics
C. To speed up billing entry
D. To generate refill reminders

Q465. What is the importance of documentation after preparing a compounded product?
A. It provides traceability for ingredients, quantities, and preparation conditions
B. It replaces pharmacist review
C. It simplifies shelf organization
D. It serves marketing purposes

Q466. Why should controlled substances be stored in a locked cabinet or secure area?
A. To reduce expiration tracking

B. To improve pharmacy design
C. To prevent diversion and ensure DEA compliance
D. To simplify workflow

Q467. Convert 0.5 liters to milliliters.
A. 500 mL
B. 50 mL
C. 5 mL
D. 0.05 mL

Q468. Why must a sterile syringe never be reused, even for the same drug preparation?
A. To prevent contamination and infection risk
B. To reduce costs
C. To maintain measurement markings
D. To improve efficiency

Q469. What should a technician do if a patient's prescription has expired refills remaining?
A. Fill it without verification
B. Dispense a partial refill
C. Override the expiration
D. Notify the pharmacist to contact the prescriber for authorization

Q470. Why should compounded non-sterile preparations be mixed with consistent technique?
A. To ensure uniform distribution of active ingredients throughout the mixture
B. To shorten preparation time
C. To create desired color uniformity
D. To reduce ingredient waste

Q471. Why must technicians verify insurance adjudication responses after claim submission?
A. To confirm payment approval and detect rejections early
B. To collect marketing data
C. To avoid pharmacist interaction
D. To modify copay values

Q472. A medication label states "Take 1 tablet QID." How many tablets per day does the patient take?
A. 4
B. 3
C. 5
D. 2

Q473. Why must pharmacy scales be calibrated regularly?
A. To avoid recordkeeping requirements
B. To ensure cosmetic uniformity
C. To maintain measurement accuracy in compounding and dispensing
D. To improve counting speed

Q474. What action should be taken when a prescription label is damaged or unreadable?
A. Reprint the label after pharmacist verification
B. Dispense it anyway
C. Handwrite the missing details
D. Discard the prescription entirely

Q475. Why is aseptic handwashing essential before sterile compounding?
A. To meet appearance standards
B. To remove microorganisms that could contaminate the preparation
C. To enhance glove comfort
D. To keep the hood area shiny

Q476. Why should technicians check for duplicate therapies in patient profiles?
A. To prevent therapeutic duplication and potential adverse reactions
B. To ensure faster workflow
C. To update patient demographics
D. To simplify inventory
Q477. A 5% w/v solution equals how many grams per 200 mL?
A. 10 g
B. 5 g
C. 15 g
D. 20 g
Q478. Why must temperature logs be maintained for pharmacy refrigerators?
A. To check humidity levels
B. To calculate monthly energy costs
C. To verify medications are stored within required stability ranges
D. To track packaging designs
Q479. Why should hazardous waste containers be color-coded and labeled clearly?
A. To prevent accidental disposal of toxic materials in regular trash
B. To simplify recycling
C. To improve storage aesthetics
D. To reduce odor
Q480. Why must sterile compounding work be performed within the direct airflow of the hood?
A. To maintain a contamination-free zone and ensure laminar airflow protection
B. To maximize visibility
C. To speed preparation
D. To improve ergonomic comfort
Q481. Why should patient allergies be reviewed before entering a new prescription?
A. To record prescription history
B. To confirm insurance status
C. To assign copay tiers
D. To prevent dispensing drugs that could cause hypersensitivity reactions
Q482. A compound requires 300 mL of solution containing 2 g of drug. What is the concentration in mg/mL?
A. 6.67 mg/mL
B. 0.67 mg/mL
C. 20 mg/mL
D. 15 mg/mL
Q483. Why must sterile gloves be disinfected with 70% isopropyl alcohol during compounding?
A. To remove surface contaminants and maintain aseptic conditions
B. To improve dexterity
C. To extend glove life
D. To dry faster between tasks
Q484. What must be verified before labeling repackaged medications?
A. Bottle size
B. Pharmacist initials
C. Prescription price
D. Drug name, strength, lot number, and expiration date
Q485. Why is documentation of compounding personnel training required?
A. To verify competency and compliance with USP standards

B. To assign work shifts
C. To monitor performance bonuses
D. To track attendance

Q486. Why must a pharmacy technician verify that the prescription date is within a valid time frame?
A. To confirm the patient's next visit
B. To update insurance copay details
C. To ensure the order is legally valid and clinically appropriate
D. To determine refill cost

Q487. Why is accurate transcription of directions critical during data entry?
A. To ensure the patient receives the correct dosing instructions
B. To save processing time
C. To record insurance details
D. To match manufacturer templates

Q488. A prescription reads: "Prednisone 10 mg — taper 4 tabs × 3 days, 3 tabs × 3 days, 2 tabs × 3 days, 1 tab × 3 days." How many tablets total?
A. 30
B. 36
C. 40
D. 32

Q489. Why should prescriptions for controlled substances include the prescriber's DEA number?
A. To verify manufacturer
B. To record patient history
C. To confirm prescriptive authority and prevent diversion
D. To identify the pharmacy

Q490. Why must reconstituted suspensions be labeled with "Shake Well"?
A. To ensure even drug distribution before each dose
B. To warn against refrigeration
C. To prevent bottle breakage
D. To reduce spillage

Q491. Convert 1.5 g of medication to milligrams.
A. 1500 mg
B. 15 mg
C. 150 mg
D. 1.5 mg

Q492. Why should technicians review drug-drug interaction alerts before processing a prescription?
A. To test software functions
B. To help identify potentially harmful medication combinations
C. To speed insurance billing
D. To update patient addresses

Q493. Why must compounded preparations be assigned a lot number?
A. To allow traceability for recalls and quality assurance
B. To track technician performance
C. To indicate expiration date
D. To record pricing

Q494. What must be confirmed before labeling a liquid prescription?
A. Refill schedule
B. Patient's insurance code
C. Manufacturer's phone number

D. Correct concentration and total volume dispensed

Q495. Why should unit-dose barcodes be scanned before administration in hospitals?

A. To confirm correct medication, dose, and patient

B. To update supply orders

C. To track billing frequency

D. To record expiration data

Q496. A patient must take 7.5 mL every 6 hours for 10 days. What total volume should be dispensed?

A. 300 mL

B. 200 mL

C. 150 mL

D. 100 mL

Q497. Why must sterile compounding areas be monitored for airborne particulates?

A. To improve room lighting

B. To maintain ISO classification and ensure environmental cleanliness

C. To adjust humidity levels

D. To increase air pressure

Q498. Why should patient profiles be updated with new prescriptions?

A. To maintain complete, current records for safety and clinical review

B. To increase database size

C. To meet marketing regulations

D. To track sales history

Q499. When compounding creams, why is geometric dilution used?

A. To enhance aroma

B. To increase cream viscosity

C. To achieve uniform distribution of potent ingredients throughout the base

D. To shorten mixing time

Q500. Why must prescriptions be checked for legally required information before filling?

A. To ensure compliance and prevent dispensing invalid orders

B. To verify patient satisfaction

C. To determine copay status

D. To reduce wait times

Answer keys and Explanations (401-500)

Q401. Answer: A

Explanation: Every compounded label must include the product name, strength, beyond-use date, and storage requirements to ensure safe and effective use. These details guide proper handling and confirm the product's stability period. Adhering to USP <795>/<797> labeling standards guarantees compliance and helps patients and healthcare providers manage compounded medications safely.

Q402. Answer: C

Explanation: Cleaning all tools and surfaces before and after compounding prevents residue from one product contaminating another. Proper hygiene ensures product purity, quality, and compliance with USP standards. This practice protects patients from adverse reactions due to cross-contamination and maintains pharmacy operational integrity during compounding processes.

Q403. Answer: A

Explanation: Beyond-use dates (BUDs) define the period during which a compounded medication maintains its potency and sterility. Assigning correct BUDs prevents patients from using expired or unstable preparations. This practice adheres to USP <795>/<797> standards and ensures patient safety by providing accurate information on the compound's stability and effectiveness.

Q404. Answer: A

Explanation: Documentation for sterile compounding must include ingredients, lot numbers, quantities used, and the preparation date. These records enable traceability, reproducibility, and quality assurance. Accurate logs ensure compliance with USP <797>, support recall management, and verify that each preparation meets safety and sterility standards for patient administration.

Q405. Answer: D

Explanation: Double verification for controlled substances confirms accuracy and prevents diversion or documentation errors. Two-person checks ensure accountability at every dispensing stage, meeting DEA and state requirements. This safeguard upholds patient safety, legal compliance, and professional integrity in handling high-risk medications with potential for abuse.

Q406. Answer: A

Explanation: When refills are exhausted, technicians must forward authorization requests to the prescriber for approval. They cannot independently approve additional refills. This process ensures medications are dispensed under continued prescriber supervision, maintaining compliance, patient safety, and regulatory integrity within the pharmacy workflow.

Q407. Answer: A

Explanation: Hazardous waste, including contaminated materials or unused drugs, must be disposed of in specifically labeled containers to prevent toxic exposure and contamination. Proper segregation complies with USP <800>, OSHA, and EPA guidelines, ensuring the safety of pharmacy staff and environmental protection from hazardous residues.

Q408. Answer: B

Explanation: Labeling repackaged unit doses with the correct drug name, strength, lot number, and expiration date ensures accurate identification and traceability. This labeling meets FDA and USP requirements and supports safety during administration. Properly labeled doses help healthcare staff verify medications before use, reducing the chance of dispensing errors.

Q409. Answer: A

Explanation: Each liquid medication may have unique viscosity or volume characteristics; using the manufacturer-provided measuring device ensures dosing accuracy. Correct measurement prevents under- or overdosing, especially for pediatric or potent liquid formulations. Accurate dosing promotes patient safety and therapeutic effectiveness across all liquid preparations.

Q410. Answer: C

Explanation: Double verification of ingredient weights ensures precise formulation and uniformity in compounded medications. Even slight deviations can impact potency or safety. Confirming each measurement supports quality assurance, reproducibility, and compliance with USP <795> guidelines, guaranteeing that the compounded product meets exact therapeutic specifications for patient safety.

Q411. Answer: A

Explanation: Proper storage labeling preserves the compounded product's stability and prevents degradation caused by heat, light, or moisture. Specific storage conditions maintain potency and safety throughout the medication's use. Clear instructions ensure patients and caregivers handle the compound correctly, complying with USP <795> and <797> standards for compounded medication quality and integrity.

Q412. Answer: A

Explanation: Inspecting vials and containers for intact seals, valid expiration dates, and absence of particles ensures sterility and product integrity. Contaminated or expired components can compromise safety or therapeutic effectiveness. This verification step upholds USP <797> standards, preventing patient exposure to unsafe sterile preparations and maintaining compounding quality assurance.

Q413. Answer: D

Explanation: Comparing the NDC number, drug name, and strength against the prescription ensures that the correct medication is selected. The NDC provides a precise identifier for drug formulation and manufacturer, reducing look-alike/sound-alike errors. This verification step supports accuracy and patient safety before tablets are counted or labeled for dispensing.

Q414. Answer: A

Explanation: The main objective of aseptic technique in sterile compounding is to prevent microbial contamination. Ensuring a sterile environment and maintaining laminar airflow integrity protect the patient from infection. Proper garbing, handwashing, and use of aseptic tools uphold USP <797> standards for sterile preparations and guarantee safe, contamination-free products.

Q415. Answer: A

Explanation: Upon identifying a prescription error, the technician must immediately stop processing and notify the pharmacist. Only the pharmacist can determine how to correct the issue. Prompt reporting prevents dispensing incorrect medications, maintaining patient safety and regulatory compliance. Technicians serve as a vital safety checkpoint in detecting potential errors early.

Q416. Answer: C

Explanation: Nitroglycerin sublingual tablets are highly sensitive to air, light, and moisture, which can reduce potency. Keeping them in their original airtight, amber glass container preserves effectiveness. Technicians must ensure these are dispensed and stored correctly, as exposure significantly decreases stability, compromising treatment for patients with angina or cardiac conditions.

Q417. Answer: A

Explanation: Detailed recordkeeping documents each step of compounding—ingredients, quantities, lot numbers, and preparation dates. This allows traceability in case of recalls, quality audits, or adverse events. Proper records demonstrate regulatory compliance, uphold professional accountability, and enable pharmacists to verify that compounding procedures were performed accurately and safely.

Q418. Answer: B

Explanation: When multiple strengths are available, technicians must confirm that the prescribed strength aligns with the SIG and prescriber's intent. Dispensing an incorrect strength can cause therapeutic failure or toxicity. Verification with the pharmacist ensures accuracy and safety, preventing dangerous dosing errors and maintaining prescriber-patient treatment integrity.

Q419. Answer: A

Explanation: Maintaining detailed, accurate dispensing logs ensures DEA compliance for controlled substances. These logs document quantities, dates, prescribers, and recipients, supporting audits and preventing diversion. Technicians assist by ensuring timely and correct record entry, upholding accountability, and meeting all legal standards for secure handling of controlled medications.

Q420. Answer: A

Explanation: Verifying patient allergies and demographic information ensures safety and proper identification before filling any prescription. This step prevents adverse drug reactions, mix-ups, or misfiled records. Technicians confirm data accuracy to create a reliable patient profile, supporting pharmacist review and ensuring safe, individualized medication therapy.

Q421. Answer: D

Explanation: Storing look-alike/sound-alike drugs apart reduces the likelihood of selection errors caused by similar names or packaging. Separation enhances identification accuracy during dispensing, aligning with ISMP recommendations for medication safety. This precaution minimizes the risk of harmful medication mix-ups, maintaining accuracy and patient protection in pharmacy operations.

Q422. Answer: A

Explanation: Before labeling, the technician must confirm the prescriber's DEA number and the number of authorized refills for controlled substances. This ensures legal dispensing compliance and prevents unauthorized refills or fraudulent prescriptions. Accurate verification aligns with DEA regulations and safeguards patients from potential misuse or medication abuse.

Q423. Answer: B

Explanation: The sterile media fill test evaluates a technician's ability to maintain aseptic technique by simulating compounding conditions using growth media. If contamination occurs, microbial growth indicates a breach. Passing the test confirms that the technician can safely prepare sterile products according to USP <797> requirements for patient protection.

Q424. Answer: A

Explanation: Single-use vials do not contain preservatives, making them prone to bacterial contamination once opened. Reusing them risks infection and violates aseptic standards. Proper disposal after one use aligns with USP <797> sterile compounding requirements and ensures patient safety by maintaining the sterility of injectable preparations.

Q425. Answer: A

Explanation: Faxed prescriptions must be verified for authenticity, including prescriber details and transmission source, before entry. Confirming validity ensures that the prescription originates from a licensed provider and complies with state and federal regulations. This verification step prevents fraudulent orders and supports safe, compliant dispensing practices.

Q426. Answer: C

Explanation: Reading back and confirming entered data ensures that all prescription details—patient name, drug, dosage, and directions—match the original order. This step minimizes transcription errors and enhances accuracy. Technicians who consistently review entries contribute significantly to dispensing safety and overall quality assurance in pharmacy practice.

Q427. Answer: A

Explanation: Hazardous drug spill kits provide essential protective equipment and materials to contain and clean accidental spills safely. Their availability ensures immediate response to contamination incidents, protecting pharmacy personnel and preventing environmental exposure. This aligns with OSHA and USP <800> safety regulations for handling hazardous pharmaceuticals.

Q428. Answer: A

Explanation: Expired medications must be removed immediately from active inventory and documented for disposal according to pharmacy policy. Dispensing expired drugs risks reduced efficacy or safety issues. Proper removal maintains product quality and compliance with FDA and pharmacy standards, ensuring only viable medications are available for dispensing.

Q429. Answer: D

Explanation: A temperature excursion alert indicates potential loss of cold-chain integrity. The technician must quarantine affected items and inform the pharmacist for assessment. This prevents dispensing compromised products and ensures compliance with manufacturer and USP storage requirements. Immediate action maintains product potency and patient safety.

Q430. Answer: A

Explanation: Visual inspection of CSPs identifies particulate matter, discoloration, or cracks in containers that could indicate contamination or instability. Detecting such issues before release prevents unsafe products from reaching patients. This mandatory quality check under USP <797> ensures sterility, safety, and product integrity in all sterile compounded preparations.

Q431. Answer: B

Explanation: Controlled substance labels must display the federal transfer warning: "Caution: Federal law prohibits the transfer of this drug to any person other than the patient for whom it was prescribed." This statement fulfills DEA requirements, reminds patients of legal restrictions, and reinforces controlled medication accountability and safe use.

Q432. Answer: A

Explanation: Verifying ingredient accuracy, concentration, and beyond-use date ensures that compounded topical creams are safe, stable, and effective. This step guarantees that all formulation details match the prescription and comply with USP <795> standards. Accurate labeling communicates essential information for proper use and patient safety.

Q433. Answer: A

Explanation: Independent double checks verify the accuracy of compounding, labeling, and calculations for high-risk preparations like chemotherapy drugs. Having two qualified individuals confirm steps independently reduces the risk of catastrophic errors. This safety measure aligns with ISMP best practices and reinforces accuracy and accountability in high-risk pharmacy operations.

Q434. Answer: C

Explanation: Any vial containing visible particles must be discarded immediately and reported to the pharmacist. Particulate contamination poses serious safety risks, including embolism or infection if administered. Discarding ensures that only sterile, uncontaminated products are used, maintaining patient safety and compliance with USP <797> quality control standards.

Q435. Answer: A

Explanation: Regular certification of airflow hoods ensures that laminar airflow and HEPA filtration effectively maintain sterile compounding environments. Certification verifies that airflow velocity and cleanliness meet USP <797> requirements. This prevents contamination, ensures technician protection, and maintains the sterile integrity of compounded medications.

Q436. Answer: A

Explanation: Verifying patient identity and date of birth ensures accurate profile creation and prevents mix-ups with other individuals. It also confirms the prescription belongs to the correct person. This step is essential to maintain legal compliance, avoid medication errors, and ensure that subsequent data entry and dispensing align with patient safety standards.

Q437. Answer: D

Explanation: An unreadable label compromises drug identification, so the technician must quarantine the bottle and alert the pharmacist. This prevents dispensing an incorrect medication, ensures inventory accuracy, and complies with pharmacy quality standards. Only the pharmacist can verify or replace questionable stock to maintain patient safety and regulatory compliance.

Q438. Answer: A

Explanation: The total daily dose equals 30 mL (10 mL × 3). Over 10 days, the patient requires 300 mL (30 × 10). Accurate calculation ensures that the correct volume is dispensed, preventing premature depletion or dosing inconsistency. Technicians apply simple multiplication to determine total quantities, ensuring therapy continuity and accurate inventory management.

Q439. Answer: B

Explanation: Handwashing, proper garbing, and disinfecting the workspace eliminate contamination risks before sterile compounding. Following this sequence ensures aseptic integrity, aligns with USP <797> standards, and prevents microbial entry. Maintaining cleanroom discipline protects both patients and pharmacy personnel, ensuring every sterile preparation meets safety and purity requirements.

Q440. Answer: A

Explanation: Only a pharmacist can clarify unclear prescriptions with the prescriber. The technician's responsibility is to recognize illegibility and halt processing. This procedure ensures accurate communication between provider and pharmacy, eliminating misinterpretation that could cause dosage or administration errors, thereby protecting patient safety.

Q441. Answer: D

Explanation: Auxiliary labels provide essential safety or usage instructions such as "Shake well" or "Avoid sunlight." They enhance patient understanding of administration, ensuring the medication is used properly and safely. Correct labeling minimizes misuse, reinforces counseling, and supports regulatory compliance by conveying key precautions directly to the patient.

Q442. Answer: A

Explanation: One gram equals 1000 milligrams; therefore, 2 grams = 2000 mg. Accurate conversions are fundamental for dosage precision in pharmacy practice. This conversion ensures the correct strength is dispensed or compounded, supporting safety in prescription fulfillment and patient therapy accuracy.

Q443. Answer: A

Explanation: Beyond-use dates ensure compounded preparations are dispensed within their proven stability period. Assigning these dates prevents use of degraded or contaminated products. Adherence to USP <795>/<797> ensures medication potency, safety, and regulatory compliance by defining when the product should be discarded.

Q444. Answer: A

Explanation: Verifying the patient's identity against the insurance card prevents billing errors and misfiled claims. This step ensures that the insurance corresponds to the correct individual's prescription profile. Proper validation supports accurate third-party processing and avoids claim denials or data mix-ups.

Q445. Answer: C

Explanation: Double-counting ensures that controlled medications match the prescription quantity exactly, preventing theft or documentation discrepancies. This accountability step upholds DEA compliance and protects against diversion. The technician's double verification guarantees accuracy and maintains trust in controlled substance handling.

Q446. Answer: A

Explanation: Each dose = 5 mL; TID = 3 × 5 = 15 mL/day. Over 10 days, total volume = 15 × 10 = 150 mL. This ensures the patient receives the complete prescribed course without running out early. Correct dosage calculations prevent under-treatment and support therapeutic consistency.

Q447. Answer: A

Explanation: Calibrated devices guarantee precise measurement of liquids and powders, ensuring consistent and accurate formulations. Using properly calibrated instruments prevents strength deviations that could affect efficacy or safety. This adherence to USP standards ensures reproducibility and maintains the integrity of compounded products.

Q448. Answer: B

Explanation: Maintaining patient confidentiality by discussing sensitive information in private prevents unauthorized disclosure and ensures compliance with HIPAA laws. Protecting data privacy fosters trust, supports ethical practice, and avoids penalties associated with breaches of patient information confidentiality.

Q449. Answer: A

Explanation: Separating look-alike medications prevents confusion during selection. Visual similarities can lead to dispensing the wrong drug or strength. Proper organization aligns with ISMP recommendations, enhancing accuracy and patient safety in high-volume pharmacy environments.

Q450. Answer: A

Explanation: 480 mg / 120 mL = 4 mg/mL. Therefore, 4 × 30 = 120 mg. Dimensional analysis ensures consistent strength relationships when scaling solutions. Correct proportional calculations prevent overdosing or underdosing and ensure uniform drug concentration per volume dispensed.

Q451. Answer: A

Explanation: Visual inspection ensures sterility and quality by identifying particulates or discoloration that indicate contamination. Detecting visual abnormalities prevents unsafe product use, complying with USP <797> and ensuring patient protection against infection or ineffective therapy.

Q452. Answer: D

Explanation: Accurate transfer documentation ensures continuity of care and prevents duplication. It includes prescription number, issue date, original pharmacy, and receiving pharmacy details. Recording this information supports legal and DEA compliance while maintaining complete patient prescription histories.

Q453. Answer: A

Explanation: Dispensing expired medications may reduce potency or cause harm. Checking expiration dates confirms product viability and therapeutic reliability. This verification ensures patient safety, aligns with FDA and state regulations, and reflects professional quality control standards in every dispensing process.

Q454. Answer: A

Explanation: "2% w/v" signifies 2 grams of solute per 100 mL of solution. Understanding percentage concentrations allows accurate preparation of solutions at correct strengths. This knowledge ensures patient doses are consistent and prevents formulation errors in compounding or dilution processes.

Q455. Answer: C

Explanation: Clean, organized compounding spaces prevent contamination between different preparations, ensuring purity and potency. Maintaining sanitary conditions aligns with USP <795> requirements, ensuring that compounded medications remain safe and effective for patients.

Q456. Answer: A

Explanation: Confirming spelling, dosage, and prescriber details ensures that the verbal prescription is entered exactly as dictated. This verification reduces transcription errors and guarantees accuracy before pharmacist approval. Precise entry is essential for legal documentation and patient safety.

Q457. Answer: A

Explanation: Unit-dose packaging provides single-use doses labeled for direct administration, minimizing preparation errors. This format enhances safety in hospitals by ensuring each patient receives the correct medication and dose. It supports barcoding systems and maintains sterile handling integrity.

Q458. Answer: A

Explanation: 4 mg/mL × 250 mL = 1000 mg. Multiplying concentration by volume provides the total active ingredient amount. This calculation ensures correct total dosage and consistent formulation, preventing dosing discrepancies when compounding or verifying liquid prescriptions.

Q459. Answer: B

Explanation: Cleaning and drying equipment prevent contamination from previous residues or moisture that could alter formulation integrity. Proper preparation ensures accurate ingredient measurement, stable product quality, and compliance with USP standards for pharmaceutical compounding.

Q460. Answer: A

Explanation: Checking for potential drug interactions during data entry allows the pharmacist to intervene early and prevent harmful combinations. Technicians play a key support role by ensuring patient profiles are updated and accurate, enabling safe clinical review before dispensing.

Q461. Answer: C

Explanation: Confirming prescription completeness, legibility, and authenticity ensures that the order meets legal and safety requirements. This prevents transcription errors and dispensing of incorrect or fraudulent prescriptions. Verification of all necessary details—such as drug, strength, directions, and prescriber signature—protects patients and maintains compliance with state and federal pharmacy regulations.

Q462. Answer: A

Explanation: Matching the quantity and SIG ensures consistency between prescribed dose, frequency, and days' supply. This logical verification prevents dispensing errors such as incorrect quantities or durations. By cross-checking these values, technicians support therapeutic accuracy and ensure that the medication supply aligns with clinical intent and insurance coverage guidelines.

Q463. Answer: B

Explanation: The total equals $(4 \times 3) + (3 \times 3) + (2 \times 3) + (1 \times 3) = 12 + 9 + 6 + 3 = 30$ tablets. Careful dosage-taper calculations ensure the entire course is dispensed accurately. Correct arithmetic prevents therapy interruption or excess supply, maintaining consistency with the prescriber's dosage schedule and patient safety.

Q464. Answer: A

Explanation: Verifying barcodes aligns the physical product with the digital prescription record, ensuring accurate dispensing. Barcode scanning prevents human error by confirming drug name, strength, and form match exactly. This step enhances accuracy, improves workflow safety, and complies with pharmacy automation quality standards.

Q465. Answer: A

Explanation: Documentation records every component used, its quantity, and the conditions under which compounding occurred. This traceability supports recalls, audits, and quality assurance. Proper records ensure accountability, reproducibility, and regulatory compliance with USP standards, maintaining the safety and integrity of compounded medications.

Q466. Answer: C

Explanation: Secure storage of controlled substances prevents unauthorized access and diversion. This measure fulfills DEA and state regulatory requirements, maintaining accountability and safety. Controlled drugs carry high abuse potential, and proper security minimizes risk, ensuring that all transactions remain traceable and compliant with legal standards.

Q467. Answer: A

Explanation: One liter equals 1000 milliliters. Multiplying 0.5×1000 yields 500 mL. Accurate unit conversions are fundamental to pharmacy calculations, ensuring precise dosing and correct solution preparation. This accuracy prevents under- or overdosing and maintains therapeutic consistency across all formulations.

Q468. Answer: A

Explanation: Reusing sterile syringes compromises aseptic integrity, introducing microbial contamination that endangers patient safety. Each syringe must remain single-use to uphold USP <797> and CDC infection control standards. Discarding after one use ensures sterility, preventing infection transmission and preserving product quality in sterile compounding.

Q469. Answer: D

Explanation: When a prescription has expired, the technician cannot dispense without renewed authorization. The pharmacist must contact the prescriber to approve continuation. This procedure ensures legal compliance, prevents unauthorized dispensing, and maintains control over ongoing therapy based on current clinical need.

Q470. Answer: A

Explanation: Consistent mixing guarantees even distribution of the active ingredient, ensuring each dose delivers the intended therapeutic effect. Poor mixing can cause potency variation, leading to under- or overdosing. Adhering to uniform technique maintains quality, accuracy, and compliance with USP <795> compounding standards.

Q471. Answer: A

Explanation: Reviewing adjudication responses ensures claims are accepted and reimbursed accurately. Detecting rejections early allows correction of errors like coverage limits or NDC mismatches. Timely resolution prevents delays in patient therapy and improves billing accuracy in the pharmacy's third-party processing workflow.

Q472. Answer: A

Explanation: "QID" means four times daily. Understanding SIG abbreviations ensures correct patient instructions and prevents dosing confusion. Proper interpretation of abbreviations is essential for accurate entry and labeling, maintaining clarity in dosage directions and supporting medication adherence.

Q473. Answer: C

Explanation: Calibration ensures scales provide accurate readings, which is critical when measuring drug ingredients or doses. Inaccurate scales may cause deviations in potency or dosing errors. Regular calibration meets USP standards, guaranteeing that all compounded or repackaged medications are consistent and therapeutically effective.

Q474. Answer: A

Explanation: If a label becomes damaged or unclear, a new label must be printed and verified by the pharmacist before dispensing. This ensures patients receive clear directions and critical warnings remain visible. Maintaining label accuracy prevents medication errors and supports professional dispensing standards.

Q475. Answer: B

Explanation: Handwashing removes microorganisms that could compromise sterile compounding environments. Following proper washing protocols ensures that gloves and gowns remain uncontaminated. This critical aseptic step aligns with USP <797> and infection control guidelines, protecting patients from harmful microbial contamination.

Q476. Answer: A

Explanation: Identifying duplicate therapies prevents patients from taking multiple medications with similar actions, reducing risk of toxicity or side effects. Technicians assist pharmacists by flagging duplicate entries during prescription processing. This safeguard promotes effective, coordinated care and avoids unnecessary medication overlap.

Q477. Answer: A

Explanation: A 5% w/v solution contains 5 g per 100 mL. For 200 mL, double the quantity to 10 g. Understanding concentration relationships allows accurate formulation of liquid medications and ensures proper therapeutic strength in compounded solutions or dilutions.

Q478. Answer: C

Explanation: Temperature logs confirm that drugs stored in refrigerators remain within the prescribed 2–8°C range for potency preservation. Daily documentation ensures compliance with USP, FDA, and manufacturer requirements, protecting medication integrity and patient safety.

Q479. Answer: A

Explanation: Color-coded labeling distinguishes hazardous waste, preventing contamination or environmental exposure. Proper segregation ensures compliance with USP <800>, OSHA, and EPA regulations. Technicians follow specific disposal guidelines to maintain a safe pharmacy environment and protect staff and public health.

Q480. Answer: A

Explanation: Working within the laminar airflow ensures the sterile product remains in the contamination-free area where air is filtered and unidirectional. This prevents microbial or particulate entry, ensuring aseptic conditions per USP <797>. Maintaining position in the airflow is critical for product sterility.

Q481. Answer: D

Explanation: Reviewing allergies ensures that medications dispensed do not trigger adverse reactions. Early detection of allergen conflicts allows pharmacists to intervene promptly and substitute safer alternatives. Maintaining updated allergy profiles safeguards patient health and supports clinical accuracy in medication selection.

Q482. Answer: A

Explanation: 2 g = 2000 mg. Divide 2000 mg ÷ 300 mL = 6.67 mg/mL. This calculation ensures correct concentration during formulation. Precision in unit conversion and proportion prevents dosing discrepancies, maintaining consistency and compliance with compounding quality standards.

Q483. Answer: A

Explanation: Disinfecting sterile gloves with alcohol eliminates potential surface microorganisms that may contaminate compounded products. This continuous aseptic measure preserves sterility throughout the process, complying with USP <797> standards. Regular sanitization reduces cross-contamination risks and ensures patient safety.

Q484. Answer: D

Explanation: Accurate labeling of repackaged drugs includes drug name, strength, lot number, and expiration date. This ensures traceability, prevents misidentification, and aligns with FDA labeling requirements. Correct labeling supports safe dispensing and compliance with recordkeeping standards in both retail and institutional pharmacy settings.

Q485. Answer: A

Explanation: Documenting training ensures that personnel performing compounding are qualified, competent, and compliant with USP <795>/<797> standards. Verified training records protect patient safety by confirming that compounding procedures are conducted correctly under aseptic and quality-controlled conditions.

Q486. Answer: C

Explanation: Prescription dates determine legal validity and therapeutic relevance. Outdated prescriptions may indicate expired therapy or a need for clinical reassessment. Verifying recency ensures compliance with federal and state regulations, particularly for controlled substances, and prevents dispensing drugs that may no longer be medically justified or safe for continued use.

Q487. Answer: A

Explanation: Precise transcription guarantees that the SIG (directions) entered matches the prescriber's original intent. Incorrect instructions could lead to underdosing, overdosing, or misuse. Ensuring accuracy protects the patient, supports pharmacist verification, and upholds legal documentation standards for safe medication dispensing.

Q488. Answer: A

Explanation: The total equals (4 × 3) + (3 × 3) + (2 × 3) + (1 × 3) = 12 + 9 + 6 + 3 = 30 tablets. Careful dosage-taper calculations ensure the entire course is dispensed accurately. Correct arithmetic prevents therapy interruption or excess supply, maintaining consistency with the prescriber's dosage schedule and patient safety.

Q489. Answer: C

Explanation: The DEA number authenticates a prescriber's authority to prescribe controlled substances. Verification prevents fraudulent or unauthorized prescriptions from being filled. Ensuring that this number is present and valid supports DEA compliance, safeguards against misuse, and maintains accountability in controlled drug dispensing.

Q490. Answer: A

Explanation: Suspensions require shaking to redistribute particles evenly for consistent dosing. Without agitation, active ingredients may settle, leading to uneven medication strength. The "Shake Well" label reinforces this essential step, ensuring therapeutic accuracy and safety with every administered dose.

Q491. Answer: A

Explanation: Since 1 g = 1000 mg, 1.5 g = 1500 mg. Converting grams to milligrams ensures correct dosage calculations and prevents strength confusion. This simple but vital step underpins accurate compounding, dispensing, and documentation, maintaining consistency across prescription and formulation records.

Q492. Answer: B

Explanation: Interaction alerts flag possible adverse combinations between prescribed and existing medications. Reviewing these ensures pharmacist awareness and intervention before dispensing. Addressing alerts proactively prevents therapeutic duplication, toxicity, or contraindicated combinations, preserving patient safety and clinical appropriateness.

Q493. Answer: A

Explanation: Assigning a lot number links each batch to its ingredient sources and compounding record. This traceability enables efficient recalls and quality checks if contamination or errors arise. Lot numbering meets USP documentation standards and ensures complete accountability for all compounded products dispensed.

Q494. Answer: D

Explanation: Ensuring correct concentration and total volume guarantees that the patient receives the proper strength and duration of therapy. Verifying these details before labeling prevents dosing inaccuracies and confusion during pharmacist verification and administration, maintaining consistency with the prescriber's intent.

Q495. Answer: A

Explanation: Barcode scanning verifies the "five rights"—right patient, drug, dose, route, and time—before administration. It eliminates manual identification errors, enhancing safety and compliance with hospital medication management systems. This process ensures precise tracking and accurate delivery of every dose to the intended patient.

Q496. Answer: A

Explanation: The patient takes 7.5 mL × 4 times daily = 30 mL/day. Over 10 days, 30 × 10 = 300 mL. Calculating total therapy volume ensures an uninterrupted regimen and precise dosing supply. Proper arithmetic confirms that patients receive sufficient medication for the prescribed treatment duration.

Q497. Answer: B

Explanation: Monitoring airborne particulates verifies that cleanrooms meet ISO cleanliness standards required by USP <797>. Regular testing ensures laminar airflow systems effectively filter contaminants. Maintaining these limits preserves aseptic conditions and protects compounded sterile preparations from microbial or particulate contamination.

Q498. Answer: A

Explanation: Updating profiles with every new prescription ensures comprehensive medication records, enabling accurate drug-interaction checks and therapy management. Up-to-date data allows pharmacists to make informed clinical decisions, minimizing errors and ensuring safe, coordinated patient care.

Q499. Answer: C

Explanation: Geometric dilution mixes small, equal portions of active ingredient with the base progressively to ensure even distribution. This method prevents concentration hot spots, guaranteeing that each dose contains consistent potency. Uniformity in compounding ensures therapeutic accuracy and product quality.

Q500. Answer: A

Explanation: Verifying required components—such as patient name, prescriber signature, and drug details—ensures prescriptions are legally valid. Missing data could make an order void or unsafe to fill. Compliance safeguards pharmacy operations and protects both patient and practitioner from regulatory violations.

Questions (501-600)

Q501. Convert 250 mg to grams.

A. 0.25 g

B. 2.5 g

C. 25 g

D. 0.025 g

Q502. Why must expired compounded preparations be removed immediately from stock?

A. To simplify labeling

B. To clear shelf space

C. To prevent dispensing products that have lost potency or stability

D. To reduce paperwork

Q503. Why should pharmacy refrigerators not be overfilled?

A. To maintain consistent airflow and temperature distribution

B. To display all labels visibly

C. To allow faster access

D. To reduce power usage

Q504. Why must label directions use clear, plain language?

A. To ensure patient understanding and safe medication use

B. To reduce printing time

C. To satisfy design standards

D. To match prescriber handwriting

Q505. A compound requires 2.4 g of drug in 120 mL of base. What is the concentration (% w/v)?

A. 2%

B. 4%

C. 1%

D. 3%

Q506. Why must a technician verify storage requirements before shelving new inventory?

A. To arrange alphabetically

B. To ensure each medication is stored under manufacturer-specified conditions

C. To facilitate promotions

D. To speed up scanning

Q507. Why must sterile compounding areas have restricted access?

A. To minimize contamination risk and maintain controlled environmental conditions

B. To store extra supplies

C. To increase workflow speed

D. To provide private counseling

Q508. Why should oral syringes be used for liquid medications in pediatric dosing?

A. To increase taste acceptance

B. To replace dosing spoons for convenience

C. To provide precise measurement and safe administration

D. To reduce labeling effort

Q509. Why must antibiotic suspensions be dispensed with a calibrated measuring device?

A. To ensure the patient measures each dose accurately at home

B. To prevent spills

C. To make bottles look complete

D. To simplify labeling

Q510. Why should compounding ingredients be verified before use?

A. To confirm identity, purity, and expiration status of each component
B. To simplify inventory tracking
C. To reduce production time
D. To test labeling printers

Q511. Why should technicians check prescription duplicates before entry?
A. To avoid dispensing the same medication twice for the same patient
B. To increase prescription count accuracy
C. To simplify billing entries
D. To save inventory space

Q512. Why must a technician confirm drug strength and dosage form before filling?
A. To record marketing data
B. To check packaging design
C. To validate insurance coverage
D. To ensure the correct product matches prescriber intent

Q513. If 1000 mL of IV fluid contains 2 g of medication, what is the concentration in mg/mL?
A. 2 mg/mL
B. 4 mg/mL
C. 0.5 mg/mL
D. 20 mg/mL

Q514. Why must a technician confirm a refill authorization before processing?
A. To speed up dispensing time
B. To ensure the refill is approved and within allowed limits
C. To maintain monthly refill quotas
D. To satisfy customer preference

Q515. Why is label verification crucial before attaching it to a container?
A. To ensure the information corresponds exactly to the prescription data
B. To reduce printing waste
C. To check label alignment
D. To improve packaging aesthetics

Q516. Why should compounded sterile products be mixed using aseptic technique?
A. To prevent microbial contamination and ensure patient safety
B. To improve product color consistency
C. To speed up workflow
D. To increase batch volume

Q517. Why must controlled substances have perpetual inventory records?
A. To predict inventory trends
B. To simplify sales reports
C. To track every transaction for compliance and accountability
D. To reduce order frequency

Q518. Convert 45 mL of a 10 mg/mL solution to total milligrams.
A. 450 mg
B. 45 mg
C. 400 mg
D. 500 mg

Q519. Why must sterile vials and ampules be disinfected before compounding?
A. To extend expiration date
B. To improve label readability
C. To enhance clarity for inspection

D. To remove surface microorganisms and prevent contamination

Q520. Why should temperature-sensitive drugs be shipped with cold packs?

A. To maintain stability and potency throughout transport
B. To meet packaging standards
C. To reduce condensation
D. To satisfy insurance carriers

Q521. Which organization publishes the list of "Error-Prone Abbreviations" to help reduce medication errors in pharmacies?

A. FDA
B. ISMP
C. NIOSH
D. CDC

Q522. A technician notices a potential look-alike/sound-alike (LASA) drug error during dispensing. What should the technician do first?

A. Continue filling and inform later
B. Hold the medication and notify the pharmacist immediately
C. Replace it with an alternative drug
D. Ignore it if dosage seems correct

Q523. Which of the following is an example of a high-alert medication?

A. Acetaminophen
B. Amoxicillin
C. Insulin
D. Ibuprofen

Q524. The use of Tall Man lettering (e.g., "predniSONE" vs. "prednisoLONE") primarily helps reduce errors associated with:

A. Similar packaging
B. Look-alike/sound-alike drug names
C. Wrong storage temperature
D. Miscalculated dosage

Q525. What is the primary goal of Continuous Quality Improvement (CQI) in pharmacy practice?

A. Punish staff for mistakes
B. Maintain compliance with DEA laws
C. Identify and correct system flaws to prevent errors
D. Reduce staffing costs

Q526. Which of the following systems allows healthcare professionals to report serious adverse drug events to the FDA?

A. MedWatch
B. VAERS
C. REMS
D. CMS

Q527. Which agency issues guidelines for handling hazardous drugs to protect healthcare workers?

A. OSHA
B. ISMP
C. NIOSH
D. DEA

Q528. What is the best immediate response if a technician discovers a near miss (an error caught before reaching the patient)?

A. Discard the record to avoid documentation

B. Report it to the pharmacist for documentation and analysis
C. Ignore since no harm occurred
D. Inform the patient

Q529. Which of the following drugs requires a Risk Evaluation and Mitigation Strategy (REMS) due to its potential for serious harm?
A. Isotretinoin
B. Metformin
C. Lisinopril
D. Acetaminophen

Q530. Which of the following best defines a medication error?
A. Harm caused by the patient not following directions
B. Any preventable event that may lead to inappropriate medication use or patient harm
C. An unavoidable reaction to a medication
D. A problem with drug manufacturing only

Q531. Which of the following actions helps prevent cross-contamination during compounding?
A. Using multi-use gloves
B. Wearing a mask only when sterile compounding
C. Labeling only after completion
D. Performing aseptic handwashing and cleaning between products

Q532. A pharmacy technician should report a potential adverse drug reaction (ADR) through which system?
A. FAERS
B. OSHA
C. CMS
D. DEA

Q533. What is the main purpose of Tall Man lettering on medication labels?
A. Reduce misinterpretation of handwritten prescriptions
B. Differentiate similar drug names visually to avoid confusion
C. Ensure proper storage labeling
D. Simplify computer entry

Q534. Which of the following would be considered a dispensing error?
A. Patient allergic reaction to a properly dispensed drug
B. Pharmacist verifying wrong strength medication
C. Physician prescribing an inappropriate drug
D. Patient failing to take medication

Q535. When cleaning areas contaminated by hazardous drugs, what type of wipes must be used?
A. Alcohol-based only
B. Dry lint-free wipes
C. Detergent and sodium hypochlorite-based wipes
D. Reusable cloth towels

Q536. Which practice supports medication adherence in patients?
A. Skipping doses when feeling better
B. Using pill organizers and reminder systems
C. Sharing medications to save cost
D. Doubling doses after missed doses

Q537. Which of the following is an example of a system-based cause of medication errors?
A. Pharmacist fatigue and understaffing
B. Patient misunderstanding

C. Incorrect drug selection by the prescriber
D. Adverse drug reaction

Q538. If a technician spills a hazardous drug, what is the first action to take?

A. Notify the pharmacist and follow the spill kit protocol
B. Wipe it up immediately with paper towels
C. Leave the area until someone else arrives
D. Dispose of it in regular trash

Q539. What is the purpose of the REMS program?

A. To regulate controlled substances
B. To ensure benefits outweigh serious risks for specific drugs
C. To monitor all over-the-counter medications
D. To enforce pharmacy technician certification

Q540. What does "root cause analysis (RCA)" help determine after a medication error?

A. The person to blame
B. The legal consequences
C. The cost of the error
D. The underlying process failures that led to the error

Q541. Which of the following is an example of a sound-alike drug pair?

A. Celexa and Celebrex
B. Lisinopril and Losartan
C. Metformin and Methadone
D. Levothyroxine and Loratadine

Q542. When a patient reports new dizziness after taking an antihypertensive, what should the technician do?

A. Tell the patient to stop taking it immediately
B. Record the symptom and notify the pharmacist
C. Recommend doubling the dose
D. Ignore the concern unless it worsens

Q543. Which organization developed the MERP (Medication Error Reporting Program)?

A. DEA
B. ISMP
C. CDC
D. CMS

Q544. Which type of error occurs if a technician labels a medication with the wrong patient name?

A. Administration error
B. Prescribing error
C. Dispensing error
D. Monitoring error

Q545. What is the purpose of using unit-dose packaging in hospitals?

A. Reduce medication costs
B. Prevent contamination and errors by providing single-use doses
C. Speed up pharmacy operations
D. Allow mixing of multiple drugs

Q546. Which of the following is a system safeguard to prevent medication errors?

A. Using handwritten logs
B. Implementing barcode verification
C. Storing LASA drugs together
D. Allowing multiple open prescriptions

Q547. Which of the following practices violates USP <797> sterile compounding standards?
A. Performing hand hygiene before gloving
B. Cleaning the hood with 70% isopropyl alcohol
C. Using sterile water for injections
D. Eating or drinking near the cleanroom
Q548. Which agency oversees REMS compliance for approved medications?
A. CDC
B. FDA
C. DEA
D. NIOSH
Q549. What should a technician do if they discover expired stock on pharmacy shelves?
A. Repackage it with a new expiration date
B. Segregate and report it to the pharmacist for disposal
C. Leave it until the next inventory
D. Dispense it if only recently expired
Q550. Which of the following is a corrective action after identifying a medication error?
A. Document, analyze, and implement system improvements
B. Destroy all pharmacy records
C. Reassign staff without reporting
D. Ignore since no harm occurred
Q551. Which statement about hazardous drug labeling is true?
A. No special label is required
B. Must include a "Caution—Hazardous Drug" label
C. Only chemotherapy drugs require labeling
D. Use a barcode label only
Q552. Which step helps prevent look-alike/sound-alike (LASA) medication errors in storage areas?
A. Storing them alphabetically
B. Storing all tablets in the same bin
C. Grouping them together for convenience
D. Physically separating and using warning labels
Q553. What is the main objective of ISMP's "Do Not Crush" list?
A. Identify drugs safe to split
B. Prevent alteration of extended-release or enteric-coated formulations
C. List drugs that taste bitter when crushed
D. Identify drugs requiring refrigeration
Q554. Which system is used to report vaccine-related adverse events?
A. FAERS
B. MedWatch
C. VAERS
D. MERP
Q555. What is the correct response to a patient receiving the wrong medication?
A. Document the error, inform the pharmacist, and follow facility policy
B. Replace the medication without reporting
C. Blame the prescriber immediately
D. Delete the error from system logs
Q556. Which statement best defines a near miss?
A. A patient harmed due to an error
B. An error detected and corrected before reaching the patient

C. A mistake that occurs repeatedly
D. A report of drug recall

Q557. What is the purpose of the MedGuide program?
A. Provide patients with information about safe and proper drug use
B. Ensure pharmacy compliance with state laws
C. Replace package inserts for professionals
D. Serve as advertising material for new drugs

Q558. Which of the following actions improves communication safety in pharmacies?
A. Using only verbal orders
B. Repeating back and verifying verbal prescriptions
C. Relying solely on memory
D. Accepting unclear handwriting without clarification

Q559. Which factor most often contributes to dispensing errors?
A. Overstaffing and multiple verification steps
B. Strict adherence to QA procedures
C. Fatigue, distractions, and high workload
D. Use of electronic health records

Q560. When documenting an incident, which detail is most essential?
A. Personal opinions about fault
B. Exact description of what occurred and when
C. Only the outcome for the patient
D. Signatures of all employees on shift

Q561. Which of the following best describes patient-centered communication in pharmacy practice?
A. Using medical jargon to display expertise
B. Providing information clearly and confirming patient understanding
C. Speaking quickly to save time
D. Avoiding patient questions during counseling

Q562. A technician receives a prescription for a medication on the ISMP "Do Not Use" abbreviation list. What should they do?
A. Fill it as written
B. Return the prescription to the patient
C. Interpret the abbreviation on their own
D. Clarify the order with the pharmacist before proceeding

Q563. When handling hazardous drugs, which personal protective equipment (PPE) is required according to NIOSH?
A. Gloves only
B. Gown, double gloves, and respirator if aerosol risk exists
C. Lab coat and mask only
D. No protection if in solid dosage form

Q564. What is the best way to reduce errors from illegible handwriting on prescriptions?
A. Use electronic prescribing systems
B. Train technicians to guess
C. Accept the order if partially legible
D. Delay filling until the next shift

Q565. If a patient receives medication intended for another person, this is an example of which error?
A. Wrong-patient error
B. Wrong-drug error
C. Wrong-strength error

D. Monitoring error

Q566. Which of the following demonstrates proper hazardous drug disposal?

A. Flushing unused medication down the sink
B. Placing waste in a yellow, leakproof, labeled container
C. Throwing it in regular trash
D. Mixing it with non-hazardous waste

Q567. Which of the following drugs should be handled as a hazardous agent per NIOSH guidelines?

A. Amlodipine
B. Lisinopril
C. Methotrexate
D. Atorvastatin

Q568. Which type of error involves dispensing the correct drug but the wrong strength?

A. Wrong-patient error
B. Wrong-strength error
C. Omission error
D. Administration error

Q569. A patient's prescription label reads "take two tablets twice daily," but the directions entered say "take one tablet daily." What type of error is this?

A. Administration error
B. Monitoring error
C. Data entry error
D. Prescribing error

Q570. Which safety practice minimizes errors during medication preparation?

A. Multitasking between prescriptions
B. Performing one prescription at a time with verification steps
C. Preparing all drugs at once for efficiency
D. Skipping verification if the order looks familiar

Q571. When a pharmacy technician checks expiration dates, which inventory method are they supporting?

A. LIFO (Last In, First Out)
B. FIFO (First In, First Out)
C. Randomized selection
D. Manual override

Q572. What is the main purpose of tall shelving separation for high-alert drugs?

A. Increase storage capacity
B. Reduce barcode use
C. Simplify technician access
D. Distinguish and isolate medications requiring extra verification

Q573. Which of the following best defines a sentinel event?

A. A minor workflow delay
B. An unexpected event causing serious harm or death
C. A patient refusing counseling
D. A system upgrade in the pharmacy

Q574. Which of the following best describes root cause analysis (RCA)?

A. Identifying underlying process failures after an error
B. Blaming the individual involved
C. Conducting random employee reviews
D. Assigning disciplinary actions

Q575. Which drug class requires independent double-checks due to high-risk potential?
A. Antihistamines
B. Anticoagulants
C. Antibiotics
D. Antacids
Q576. When a pharmacy receives a drug recall notice, what should the technician do first?
A. Continue using the drug until stock runs out
B. Segregate recalled stock and notify the pharmacist
C. Ignore it if patients report no issues
D. Dispose of it immediately without verification
Q577. Which of the following drugs should be stored in a hazardous drug area under USP <800>?
A. Levothyroxine
B. Hydrochlorothiazide
C. Simvastatin
D. Doxorubicin
Q578. Which safety measure is required when compounding hazardous drugs?
A. Use of a containment primary engineering control (C-PEC)
B. Mixing in an open-air workspace
C. Wearing a single pair of gloves only
D. Avoiding negative pressure ventilation
Q579. Which of the following represents proper error reporting culture?
A. Fear-based punishment
B. Encouraging staff to report without blame
C. Ignoring minor incidents
D. Limiting reports to serious harm cases
Q580. Which of the following practices supports infection control in sterile compounding?
A. Wearing artificial nails or jewelry
B. Using sterile gloves and aseptic handwashing
C. Handling food in the buffer area
D. Avoiding gowning to save time
Q581. Which of the following would most likely prevent medication mix-ups in automated dispensing cabinets (ADCs)?
A. Allowing multiple drugs per bin
B. Stocking only generic medications
C. Labeling and separating LASA drugs in distinct drawers
D. Disabling barcode verification
Q582. Which of the following should be included when documenting a medication error?
A. The staff member's opinion about the cause
B. A factual account of the event, time, and actions taken
C. Personal blame assignments
D. Future disciplinary plans
Q583. Which of the following safety programs is focused on preventing workplace exposure to hazardous substances?
A. ISMP MERP
B. NIOSH hazardous drug handling guidelines
C. FDA MedWatch
D. CDC Immunization Initiative
Q584. What is the most critical step before releasing a filled prescription to the patient?

A. Counting the tablets again
B. Placing it in a bag
C. Printing the receipt
D. Final verification by the pharmacist

Q585. A technician receives a prescription with illegible handwriting and uncertain dosing. What is the safest action?
A. Ask the patient what the doctor meant
B. Guess the intended dose
C. Hold the order and alert the pharmacist for clarification
D. Fill the most common strength

Q586. Which of the following defines a Category A medication error according to NCC MERP?
A. An error that reached the patient but caused no harm
B. Circumstances with potential for error but no occurrence
C. An error causing temporary harm
D. An error requiring intervention to sustain life

Q587. What should a technician do if they notice a coworker repeatedly bypassing safety checks?
A. Ignore it to avoid conflict
B. Report the behavior confidentially to a supervisor or pharmacist
C. Confront them in front of patients
D. Do nothing unless an error occurs

Q588. Which infection control measure must always be performed before entering the cleanroom?
A. Handwashing with antimicrobial soap and warm water
B. Putting on gloves first
C. Spraying hands with alcohol only
D. Touching supplies to test sterility

Q589. A technician accidentally drops sterile syringes on the cleanroom floor. What should they do?
A. Reuse them if the wrapper is intact
B. Discard them as contaminated and replace with new ones
C. Wipe them with alcohol and reuse
D. Set them aside for later cleaning

Q590. Which of the following is an example of a communication-related medication error?
A. Misreading a prescriber's abbreviation
B. Using expired medication
C. Incorrect storage temperature
D. Overfilling a capsule

Q591. Which organization develops USP <795>, <797>, and <800> standards?
A. CDC
B. FDA
C. United States Pharmacopeia (USP)
D. ISMP

Q592. Which measure best prevents dose miscalculations during compounding?
A. Using mental math for speed
B. Double-checking all calculations independently
C. Skipping rechecks if confident
D. Estimating based on previous batches

Q593. Which is the most accurate way to identify the correct patient in a healthcare setting?
A. Ask for name and verify date of birth
B. Recognize the patient's face

C. Verify insurance provider
D. Ask for address only

Q594. Which step ensures traceability when managing controlled substances?
A. Documenting every receipt, use, and waste
B. Verifying stock weekly only
C. Allowing shared passwords for logging
D. Skipping DEA log updates

Q595. Which of the following represents an error of omission?
A. Administering a higher dose than prescribed
B. Recording incorrect administration time
C. Giving the wrong patient a correct drug
D. Failing to administer a scheduled medication

Q596. What is the best way to minimize environmental contamination when compounding sterile products?
A. Keep airflow blocked by supplies
B. Maintain unobstructed airflow in the hood
C. Store personal items near the workspace
D. Reuse syringes for multiple products

Q597. What should be done when a pharmacy refrigerator temperature exceeds safe limits?
A. Ignore it unless drugs look damaged
B. Notify the pharmacist and quarantine affected medications
C. Reset it without recording
D. Continue dispensing as normal

Q598. Why is continuous education and competency assessment important for technicians?
A. It fulfills a state board formality
B. It only benefits management
C. It ensures maintained proficiency in safety and quality standards
D. It reduces pharmacist oversight

Q599. Which federal agency manages the FAERS database for adverse drug event reporting?
A. CDC
B. DEA
C. FDA
D. CMS

Q600. Which principle defines a "just culture" in pharmacy safety?
A. Zero tolerance for all errors
B. Balancing accountability with non-punitive error reporting
C. Allowing staff to ignore policies
D. Punishing every error equally

Answer keys and Explanations (501-600)

Q501. Answer: A

Explanation: Dividing 250 mg ÷ 1000 = 0.25 g. Accurate conversion between milligrams and grams guarantees correct dosage formulation and labeling. Precision in unit translation prevents serious medication errors, supporting the technician's role in ensuring dosage integrity and accuracy during dispensing or compounding.

Q502. Answer: C

Explanation: Expired compounds may degrade chemically or microbiologically, compromising safety and efficacy. Prompt removal ensures that only potent, stable medications reach patients. This process aligns with USP <795>/<797> stability standards and supports pharmacy quality assurance and patient protection.

Q503. Answer: A

Explanation: Overfilling blocks air circulation, creating temperature variations that can destabilize medications. Proper spacing ensures uniform cooling within the 2–8 °C range, maintaining potency. Monitoring organization and load prevents thermal pockets, preserving drug integrity in line with USP storage guidelines.

Q504. Answer: A

Explanation: Using clear, non-technical directions improves patient comprehension, adherence, and safety. Plain language eliminates confusion caused by complex medical terms, reducing risk of misuse. Effective communication through labeling supports patient empowerment and aligns with health literacy principles in pharmacy practice.

Q505. Answer: A

Explanation: Percent w/v = (grams ÷ mL) × 100 = (2.4 ÷ 120) × 100 = 2%. Calculating concentration ensures that compounded medications meet prescribed strength requirements. Correct computations maintain dosage accuracy and product uniformity, supporting professional compounding standards.

Q506. Answer: B

Explanation: Storing drugs under correct conditions (temperature, light, humidity) preserves potency and stability. Verifying manufacturer guidelines ensures products maintain therapeutic effectiveness throughout their shelf life. Proper storage is integral to pharmaceutical quality control and patient safety.

Q507. Answer: A

Explanation: Limiting access to authorized, garbed personnel prevents introduction of contaminants and upholds environmental control within cleanrooms. Restricted entry maintains ISO air standards required by USP <797>, ensuring sterile conditions and protecting compounded preparations from microbial contamination.

Q508. Answer: C

Explanation: Oral syringes measure small volumes accurately, crucial for pediatric or concentrated liquid medications. They prevent dosing errors associated with household spoons, ensuring each administration is precise. This accuracy promotes therapeutic safety and adherence for sensitive pediatric patients.

Q509. Answer: A

Explanation: Including a calibrated device guarantees that patients measure correct doses, avoiding under- or overdosing. Accurate measurement sustains therapeutic levels, ensuring effective infection treatment. This standard supports patient education and safe home administration practices.

Q510. Answer: A

Explanation: Verifying ingredient identity, purity, and expiration ensures compounded products meet safety and potency standards. Using incorrect or expired substances compromises stability and effectiveness. This verification step maintains compliance with USP <795>/<797> and guarantees that each compounded medication meets pharmaceutical quality requirements.

Q511. Answer: A

Explanation: Checking for duplicates prevents duplicate therapy, which can cause overdosing or adverse effects. Reviewing patient profiles ensures that repeat entries are detected early. Preventing duplicate dispensing maintains safety, reduces medication waste, and ensures proper continuity of treatment as per prescriber intent.

Q512. Answer: D

Explanation: Confirming drug strength and dosage form guarantees that the dispensed product aligns precisely with the prescriber's order. Many drugs exist in multiple strengths and formulations, making verification critical to avoid therapeutic errors. This check protects patients and ensures the prescription fulfills exact clinical requirements.

Q513. Answer: A

Explanation: Two grams equals 2000 mg. Dividing 2000 mg by 1000 mL gives 2 mg/mL. Concentration calculations confirm that compounded IV solutions provide the prescribed strength. Ensuring precise proportions prevents subtherapeutic dosing or toxicity, supporting correct infusion preparation and patient safety.

Q514. Answer: B

Explanation: Confirming refill authorization ensures the prescriber has approved continued therapy and that the refill falls within the legal and insurance parameters. Unauthorized refills may violate regulations or endanger patients. This verification step maintains compliance and safe, controlled medication use.

Q515. Answer: A

Explanation: Verifying labels guarantees that patient details, drug name, and directions match the prescription. Labeling errors can lead to serious administration mistakes. Accuracy at this stage prevents dispensing confusion, supports pharmacist final checks, and ensures regulatory compliance for prescription integrity and safety.

Q516. Answer: A

Explanation: Aseptic technique ensures no microorganisms enter sterile compounded preparations. Maintaining sterility through hand hygiene, cleanroom protocols, and laminar airflow prevents infection risk and product contamination. This process aligns with USP <797> requirements and is fundamental for ensuring sterile, safe compounded medications.

Q517. Answer: C

Explanation: Perpetual inventory records maintain a continuous account of all controlled substance movements—receipts, dispensing, and returns. This ongoing record ensures DEA compliance, deters diversion, and allows immediate discrepancy detection. It upholds transparency and integrity in managing high-risk medications.

Q518. Answer: A

Explanation: Multiplying 45 mL × 10 mg/mL = 450 mg. This proportional calculation confirms total drug content for dispensing or compounding accuracy. Mastering simple multiplication ensures correct formulation, therapeutic consistency, and prevention of dosing errors in liquid medication preparation.

Q519. Answer: D

Explanation: Disinfecting vial stoppers and ampule necks with sterile alcohol removes surface microbes that could contaminate compounded solutions. This step preserves aseptic conditions and complies with USP <797> protocols. Proper disinfection protects product sterility and ensures patient safety from potential infection.

Q520. Answer: A

Explanation: Temperature-sensitive drugs require controlled shipping to remain effective. Cold packs keep products within their specified temperature range during transit, preventing degradation. This step ensures that biologicals, vaccines, and similar drugs retain full potency upon arrival, aligning with manufacturer and USP storage standards.

Q521. Answer: B

Explanation: The Institute for Safe Medication Practices (ISMP) publishes the "Error-Prone Abbreviations List," guiding healthcare workers to avoid unsafe abbreviations like "U" for units. This promotes standardized communication, reducing confusion that could lead to dosage errors. The FDA supports labeling accuracy but not this specific list, while NIOSH focuses on hazardous drugs and the CDC on infectious disease control, not abbreviations.

Q522. Answer: B

Explanation: Pharmacy technicians must immediately pause dispensing and alert the pharmacist upon detecting potential LASA confusion. Early intervention prevents dispensing of the wrong medication. Continuing to fill or substituting independently exceeds technician authority. Immediate pharmacist review ensures safety verification before release, aligning with ISMP and quality assurance standards for medication error prevention in pharmacy practice.

Q523. Answer: C

Explanation: Insulin is classified as a high-alert medication because minor errors in dosing or timing can lead to life-threatening hypoglycemia or hyperglycemia. ISMP lists insulin, anticoagulants, and opioids among drugs requiring extra precautions. Acetaminophen and ibuprofen, though common, have wider safety margins, and amoxicillin errors rarely cause immediate life-threatening consequences, making insulin the most critical for double verification.

Q524. Answer: B

Explanation: Tall Man lettering differentiates similar drug names to prevent LASA confusion in prescribing and dispensing. Highlighting portions of names like "hydrOXYzine" and "hydrALAZINE" helps staff distinguish between distinct medications. Packaging and temperature errors stem from different issues, not name confusion. This strategy is endorsed by the FDA and ISMP as part of standardized medication safety initiatives.

Q525. Answer: C

Explanation: CQI aims to systematically analyze workflow processes and correct system-based weaknesses that contribute to medication errors. It fosters a non-punitive culture that encourages error reporting to improve safety and efficiency. DEA compliance and staffing are operational concerns, not CQI's focus. CQI's proactive model enhances patient care through ongoing evaluation and implementation of safer practices.

Q526. Answer: A

Explanation: The FDA's MedWatch program enables healthcare professionals and consumers to report adverse drug events, product quality problems, or medication errors. The information supports post-marketing surveillance and regulatory actions. VAERS is specific to vaccine-related events, REMS ensures safe use of high-risk drugs, and CMS handles healthcare reimbursement, not medication safety reporting, making MedWatch the correct system.

Q527. Answer: C

Explanation: The National Institute for Occupational Safety and Health (NIOSH) sets standards for safe handling of hazardous drugs, including chemotherapy agents. Their guidelines prevent occupational exposure by recommending PPE, engineering controls, and proper disposal. OSHA enforces workplace safety laws but follows NIOSH's recommendations. DEA manages controlled substances, and ISMP focuses on medication safety systems, not hazardous handling.

Q528. Answer: B

Explanation: Even if no harm occurs, near misses must be reported to the pharmacist for proper documentation and quality review. This information helps identify system vulnerabilities and prevents future errors. Ignoring or hiding incidents defeats continuous improvement goals. Patient notification is unnecessary if the medication was not dispensed, as focus should remain on internal safety enhancement.

Q529. Answer: A

Explanation: Isotretinoin has a REMS program called iPLEDGE, which ensures patients understand and comply with strict pregnancy prevention requirements due to its high teratogenic risk. REMS programs mitigate risks of severe adverse effects by requiring monitoring, education, or registration. Metformin, lisinopril, and acetaminophen, while potentially harmful, are not subject to mandatory REMS controls.

Q530. Answer: B

Explanation: A medication error is defined by the NCC MERP as any preventable event that could lead to inappropriate medication use or harm. It includes errors in prescribing, dispensing, administration, or monitoring. Noncompliance and manufacturing defects are separate issues. This definition emphasizes prevention and system improvement rather than assigning blame to individuals.

Q531. Answer: D

Explanation: Proper handwashing, surface disinfection, and equipment cleaning between compounding sessions minimize contamination and product mix-ups. Reusing gloves or partial protective equipment risks spreading contaminants. Labeling alone doesn't ensure cleanliness. Cross-contamination control aligns with USP <795> and <797> standards, emphasizing aseptic practices in sterile and non-sterile compounding to maintain product purity and patient safety.

Q532. Answer: A

Explanation: The FDA Adverse Event Reporting System (FAERS) collects and analyzes post-marketing reports of suspected ADRs. Data supports ongoing drug safety evaluation. OSHA governs workplace safety, CMS manages healthcare funding, and DEA enforces controlled substance regulations. Technicians assist pharmacists in reporting through FAERS to ensure continued medication safety and regulatory oversight.

Q533. Answer: B

Explanation: Tall Man lettering highlights distinctive parts of drug names (e.g., hydrOXYzine vs. hydrALAZINE) to prevent confusion between look-alike/sound-alike drugs. It's a visual safety tool endorsed by ISMP and FDA. It doesn't address handwriting interpretation or storage labeling directly, nor is it designed for data entry simplification. Its sole goal is preventing selection and dispensing errors.

Q534. Answer: B

Explanation: A dispensing error occurs when the correct prescription is filled incorrectly — such as providing the wrong strength, dosage form, or medication. Physician prescribing errors occur before dispensing, and patient noncompliance happens afterward. Allergic reactions are adverse events, not errors. Dispensing errors highlight the importance of final verification before medication release to patients.

Q535. Answer: C

Explanation: NIOSH and USP <800> recommend detergent and sodium hypochlorite (bleach)-based wipes for cleaning hazardous drug residues, ensuring chemical deactivation and surface decontamination. Alcohol wipes alone don't neutralize hazardous substances, while reusable cloths risk recontamination. Proper cleaning reduces exposure risks to healthcare personnel and maintains compliance with safe handling standards.

Q536. Answer: B

Explanation: Pill organizers, smartphone reminders, and pharmacist counseling significantly enhance medication adherence. These tools help patients maintain correct dosing schedules and avoid omissions. Skipping, sharing, or doubling doses increases risk of treatment failure or toxicity. Adherence promotion improves therapeutic outcomes and patient safety, aligning with pharmacy technicians' supportive role in patient care management.

Q537. Answer: A

Explanation: System-based causes stem from workflow or environmental issues such as staff fatigue, inadequate verification steps, or poor communication. These reflect organizational deficiencies, not individual incompetence. Patient misunderstanding is a user-related factor, while prescriber selection errors occur upstream. Recognizing system-based causes helps implement process improvements to prevent future medication errors efficiently.

Q538. Answer: A

Explanation: The technician must immediately notify the pharmacist and follow the spill response protocol using a designated hazardous drug spill kit. This includes PPE, absorbent materials, and disposal containers to safely neutralize contamination. Paper towels or standard trash disposal violate NIOSH and USP <800> safety requirements, risking exposure to staff and contamination of work areas.

Q539. Answer: B

Explanation: The FDA's Risk Evaluation and Mitigation Strategies (REMS) ensures that medications with severe safety risks, like clozapine or isotretinoin, are used safely under controlled conditions. REMS may include training, patient registries, or monitoring. It's unrelated to controlled substances or technician credentialing. Its purpose is protecting patients while maintaining drug access where benefits exceed risks.

Q540. Answer: D

Explanation: Root Cause Analysis (RCA) identifies systemic failures—such as miscommunication, workflow breakdowns, or inadequate checks—that caused a medication error. It emphasizes learning and prevention, not punishment. RCA's findings drive improvements in training, labeling, and verification systems. Evaluating underlying processes ensures safety culture advancement and sustained reduction of medication errors in practice.

Q541. Answer: A

Explanation: Celexa (citalopram) and Celebrex (celecoxib) are classic sound-alike medications often confused during prescribing or dispensing due to phonetic similarity. Both drugs treat very different conditions—depression versus pain/inflammation. ISMP lists this pair as high-risk for LASA errors. The other pairs differ more in spelling or use, making them less frequently confused in clinical environments.

Q542. Answer: B

Explanation: Pharmacy technicians must document and promptly notify the pharmacist about any adverse effects reported by patients, such as dizziness from antihypertensives. The pharmacist can assess drug-related causes and determine appropriate actions. Technicians cannot modify therapy or advise discontinuation. Immediate documentation supports pharmacovigilance, patient counseling, and accurate reporting through systems like MedWatch or FAERS.

Q543. Answer: B

Explanation: The Institute for Safe Medication Practices (ISMP) created the Medication Error Reporting Program (MERP) to collect and analyze voluntary reports of medication errors. Data from MERP improves systems and processes to prevent recurrence. The DEA oversees controlled substances, the CDC focuses on public health surveillance, and CMS handles healthcare payment systems, not medication error reporting.

Q544. Answer: C

Explanation: Labeling a medication for the wrong patient constitutes a dispensing error, as the mistake occurs within the pharmacy before administration. Such errors can lead to severe harm if uncorrected. Administration errors occur during medication delivery to the patient, prescribing errors originate with the provider, and monitoring errors relate to failure to observe treatment response or side effects.

Q545. Answer: B

Explanation: Unit-dose packaging delivers a single medication dose in a sealed, clearly labeled container, minimizing contamination and administration errors. It ensures correct identification, protects stability, and reduces cross-contamination risk. While efficiency and cost management are benefits, the primary purpose is enhancing patient safety and accuracy in dispensing and administration, especially in institutional settings.

Q546. Answer: B

Explanation: Barcode verification systems ensure correct medication selection, strength, and patient matching, significantly reducing dispensing and administration errors. It cross-checks data electronically against the prescription order. Handwritten logs increase transcription risk, and storing LASA drugs together promotes confusion. Barcode systems are part of modern quality assurance technology promoting safety and traceability in pharmacy operations.

Q547. Answer: D

Explanation: USP <797> strictly prohibits eating, drinking, or storing food in or near sterile compounding areas to prevent contamination. Personnel must maintain aseptic technique, clean work surfaces with 70% isopropyl alcohol, and use sterile materials. Even minor breaches like food or beverages in clean zones compromise product sterility and violate infection control requirements.

Q548. Answer: B

Explanation: The Food and Drug Administration (FDA) is responsible for developing, approving, and monitoring Risk Evaluation and Mitigation Strategies (REMS) to ensure safe medication use for high-risk drugs. Manufacturers must comply with FDA-mandated REMS requirements. DEA governs controlled substances, CDC manages public health programs, and NIOSH focuses on workplace safety standards, not REMS oversight.

Q549. Answer: B

Explanation: Expired medications must be removed immediately, isolated from active stock, and reported to the pharmacist for proper disposal or return per FDA and state board regulations. Repurposing or extending expiration dates violates safety and compliance laws. Dispensing expired drugs risks reduced potency or contamination. Proper stock rotation (FIFO) prevents future occurrences.

Q550. Answer: A

Explanation: Following a medication error, pharmacies must document, review, and apply corrective actions as part of a continuous quality improvement process. This includes analyzing causes, revising procedures, and retraining staff if necessary. Destroying records or avoiding reports prevents learning opportunities. Even harm-free events must be analyzed to strengthen safety measures and prevent recurrence.

Q551. Answer: B

Explanation: All hazardous drugs—chemotherapeutic or otherwise—must display a "Caution—Hazardous Drug" label per NIOSH and USP <800> requirements. This warning ensures proper handling, storage, and disposal precautions. Limiting labels to chemotherapy drugs or using generic barcodes omits critical safety information, increasing risk of exposure or contamination during transport and administration.

Q552. Answer: D

Explanation: To minimize LASA confusion, pharmacies must separate similar-sounding or -looking drugs and apply auxiliary warning labels. ISMP recommends distinct storage locations, Tall Man lettering, and color-coded bins. Alphabetical or grouped storage increases error potential, while generic bin placement eliminates visual differentiation, risking accidental selection during dispensing.

Q553. Answer: B

Explanation: The ISMP "Do Not Crush" list warns against crushing medications that are extended-release, enteric-coated, or otherwise altered by mechanical manipulation, as it can lead to dose dumping or loss of protection. These designations preserve pharmacokinetic integrity. Crushing safe or coated tablets could cause toxicity or reduced efficacy, compromising medication safety and therapeutic outcomes.

Q554. Answer: C

Explanation: The Vaccine Adverse Event Reporting System (VAERS), jointly managed by the FDA and CDC, collects reports of post-vaccination side effects or errors. Data helps monitor vaccine safety and identify rare reactions. FAERS handles other drug-related events, MedWatch reports general adverse drug effects, and MERP focuses on medication error prevention rather than vaccine monitoring.

Q555. Answer: A

Explanation: Upon identifying a wrong-medication error, the technician must immediately notify the pharmacist, document the incident, and follow established reporting protocols. Transparency ensures appropriate corrective action and patient notification. Concealing errors or assigning blame prevents learning and violates pharmacy regulations. Prompt communication supports accountability and protects patient safety.

Q556. Answer: B

Explanation: A near miss refers to a potential medication error intercepted before it affects the patient, such as catching a wrong dose during verification. Reporting near misses helps identify system vulnerabilities and improve safety protocols. Unlike actual errors causing harm, near misses highlight prevention success but still require documentation for continuous process improvement and staff education.

Q557. Answer: A

Explanation: Medication Guides (MedGuides) are FDA-approved patient education documents that accompany certain high-risk drugs. They explain safe use, potential side effects, and risk mitigation strategies in plain language. They supplement, not replace, professional labeling. Their goal is to empower patients with critical safety information, promoting adherence and preventing misuse or serious adverse effects.

Q558. Answer: B

Explanation: "Read-back or repeat-back verification" ensures accuracy when receiving verbal orders by confirming patient, drug, and dosage details aloud. It prevents transcription and interpretation errors. Relying on memory or unclear handwriting increases risk of miscommunication and medication errors. Effective communication protocols form a core component of medication safety culture in pharmacy operations.

Q559. Answer: C

Explanation: Human factors—especially fatigue, interruptions, and excessive workload—are leading contributors to dispensing errors. These conditions reduce attention to detail and verification accuracy. QA procedures and EHR systems, when properly used, lower error rates, not increase them. Addressing environmental factors through staffing, workflow design, and rest breaks enhances focus and safety.

Q560. Answer: B

Explanation: Accurate documentation must include a clear, factual description of what occurred, when, and how the error or event was discovered. Objective reporting enables proper analysis and system improvement. Opinions or blame reduce the usefulness of reports. Recording exact times, drug details, and corrective actions supports regulatory compliance and safety auditing processes.

Q561. Answer: B

Explanation: Patient-centered communication emphasizes using simple, clear language, verifying understanding with the teach-back method, and encouraging questions. It builds trust and supports medication adherence by ensuring patients fully comprehend directions. Medical jargon and rushed communication increase confusion and noncompliance. Active listening and feedback confirm that counseling achieves comprehension, which is essential for safe medication use.

Q562. Answer: D

Explanation: When encountering unsafe abbreviations (e.g., "U" for units or "QD" for daily), the technician must consult the pharmacist to clarify the order before processing. Misinterpreting abbreviations risks dangerous dosing errors. ISMP's "Do Not Use" list promotes standardization and safety by eliminating ambiguous shorthand that could lead to incorrect medication administration or patient harm.

Q563. Answer: B

Explanation: NIOSH mandates double chemotherapy-rated gloves, a disposable gown, and a respirator if aerosols or powders may be released. Even solid dosage forms can generate residues that pose exposure risks. PPE protects technicians from carcinogenic, teratogenic, or toxic effects. Simple lab coats or single gloves are insufficient, violating USP <800> and NIOSH handling protocols.

Q564. Answer: A

Explanation: Electronic prescribing (e-prescribing) eliminates interpretation errors caused by illegible handwriting by transmitting prescriptions directly from prescribers to pharmacies. It improves clarity, reduces transcription errors, and enhances patient safety. Guessing or delaying orders violates policy, and partial interpretation risks serious harm. E-prescribing is an essential advancement in medication safety and workflow efficiency.

Q565. Answer: A

Explanation: Dispensing or administering medication to the wrong individual is a wrong-patient error, a serious safety breach often caused by verification lapses. Technicians must confirm two unique patient identifiers (e.g., name and date of birth) before dispensing. This protocol prevents mix-ups and aligns with ISMP and Joint Commission safety standards for patient identification verification.

Q566. Answer: B

Explanation: Hazardous drug waste must be placed in yellow, puncture-resistant, leakproof containers clearly labeled "Hazardous Drug Waste." These containers comply with EPA, NIOSH, and USP <800> standards to prevent environmental contamination and occupational exposure. Flushing or mixing waste with regular trash violates hazardous waste regulations and endangers both staff and the community.

Q567. Answer: C

Explanation: Methotrexate is listed by NIOSH as a hazardous antineoplastic agent due to its carcinogenic, teratogenic, and organ toxicity risks. It requires PPE, containment devices, and disposal precautions under USP <800>. Amlodipine, lisinopril, and atorvastatin do not pose these hazards and can be handled with standard precautions, making methotrexate the correct answer.

Q568. Answer: B

Explanation: A wrong-strength error occurs when the correct drug and patient are selected, but the dosage strength dispensed differs from what was prescribed. It often results from shelf mix-ups or labeling mistakes. Technicians must verify strength during every step of the filling process to ensure accuracy. Omission and administration errors involve different stages of medication handling.

Q569. Answer: C

Explanation: A data entry error happens when prescription details are incorrectly typed into the system, leading to mismatched directions on the label. This discrepancy can result in underdosing or overdosing. Technicians must double-check entries and cross-verify against the original prescription to prevent medication errors caused by inaccurate transcription or typographical mistakes.

Q570. Answer: B

Explanation: Preparing one prescription at a time ensures focused attention and accuracy. It allows proper verification of the drug, dose, and patient information before proceeding to the next task. Multitasking and skipping checks invite distractions and increase error risk. Standardizing a stepwise workflow supports safety, consistency, and reduced cognitive overload during dispensing.

Q571. Answer: B

Explanation: The FIFO method ensures older stock is used before newer stock by rotating inventory so that medications closest to expiration are dispensed first. This minimizes waste and prevents accidental use of expired drugs. The LIFO method is incompatible with expiration control, while random selection lacks structure. FIFO supports both compliance and cost-effective inventory management.

Q572. Answer: D

Explanation: Storing high-alert drugs on separate, clearly marked shelves prevents confusion and encourages additional verification steps before dispensing. This physical segregation minimizes mix-ups and reinforces alertness among staff. Increasing capacity or simplifying access doesn't enhance safety; instead, separation supports ISMP-recommended storage protocols for medications with significant potential for patient harm if misused.

Q573. Answer: B

Explanation: A sentinel event is an unexpected occurrence that results in death, serious physical or psychological injury, or risk thereof. The Joint Commission requires investigation and Root Cause Analysis for all sentinel events to prevent recurrence. They highlight severe breakdowns in safety systems, demanding prompt corrective action. Minor delays or workflow issues don't qualify as sentinel events.

Q574. Answer: A

Explanation: Root Cause Analysis (RCA) focuses on identifying system-level causes behind medication errors to prevent recurrence. It emphasizes process improvement rather than punishment. RCA investigates workflow gaps, communication failures, or environmental factors contributing to the incident. This method promotes learning and accountability by improving systems, aligning with continuous quality improvement goals in healthcare.

Q575. Answer: B

Explanation: Anticoagulants like warfarin and heparin are high-alert medications requiring independent double verification by two qualified personnel before dispensing or administration. Even small dosage errors can cause fatal bleeding or thrombosis. ISMP mandates special handling, labeling, and monitoring protocols. Other classes like antihistamines or antacids have wider therapeutic margins and are not subject to double-check requirements.

Q576. Answer: B

Explanation: Upon receiving a recall notice, technicians must isolate affected products, halt dispensing, and inform the pharmacist immediately. The pharmacist then verifies the recall classification (I, II, or III) and determines whether patient notification is required. Unverified disposal or continued use violates FDA recall procedures. Accurate documentation and segregation ensure safety and compliance.

Q577. Answer: D

Explanation: Doxorubicin, a cytotoxic chemotherapy agent, must be stored in a designated hazardous drug containment area per USP <800>. This protects staff from exposure through aerosols or contact. These areas feature negative pressure and externally vented hoods. Routine drugs like levothyroxine or statins lack such requirements. Proper containment is crucial for maintaining occupational safety.

Q578. Answer: A

Explanation: Hazardous drug compounding must occur within a Containment Primary Engineering Control (C-PEC), such as a biological safety cabinet or compounding aseptic containment isolator. These devices provide HEPA filtration and negative pressure to prevent exposure. Open-air compounding or insufficient PPE violates USP <800> standards, increasing risk of contamination and occupational harm.

Q579. Answer: B

Explanation: A non-punitive, open reporting culture encourages all staff to report actual and near-miss events, promoting transparency and system improvement. Fear of punishment discourages reporting and conceals hazards. Continuous quality improvement relies on open communication and learning from all incidents, regardless of severity, to strengthen processes and prevent future medication errors.

Q580. Answer: B

Explanation: Sterile compounding requires aseptic handwashing and use of sterile gloves, gowns, and hair covers to prevent microbial contamination. Jewelry and artificial nails harbor bacteria and are prohibited in cleanrooms. Handling food or skipping gowning compromises sterility. Following USP <797> infection control standards ensures compounded preparations remain safe for patient use.

Q581. Answer: C

Explanation: Separating look-alike/sound-alike (LASA) drugs into distinct, clearly labeled ADC drawers reduces selection errors. Combined with barcode verification, this prevents wrong-drug dispensing. Placing multiple drugs in the same bin or disabling barcodes increases risk. Proper ADC configuration, double verification, and staff training maintain system integrity and ensure safe medication administration in institutional settings.

Q582. Answer: B

Explanation: Documentation must remain factual and objective, including the exact event description, time, and corrective steps taken. Opinions, blame, or disciplinary notes compromise report accuracy and prevent learning. Factual reporting supports Root Cause Analysis (RCA) and continuous quality improvement. Accurate records also ensure compliance with regulatory agencies and legal standards for medication safety.

Q583. Answer: B

Explanation: The NIOSH hazardous drug handling guidelines focus on preventing worker exposure to toxic agents during preparation, storage, and disposal. These protocols define PPE requirements, engineering controls, and facility design under USP <800>. ISMP MERP addresses medication error reporting, while MedWatch covers drug adverse events. NIOSH specifically safeguards healthcare workers through exposure prevention practices.

Q584. Answer: D

Explanation: A pharmacist must perform final verification of all prescriptions before release, ensuring accuracy in drug, dose, patient, and labeling. This step confirms safety and legal compliance. Technicians handle preparation, but the pharmacist's professional judgment is required to detect potential interactions, contraindications, or errors. Skipping this verification violates federal and state pharmacy regulations.

Q585. Answer: C

Explanation: Technicians must not interpret unclear prescriptions. The correct response is to immediately notify the pharmacist, who contacts the prescriber for clarification. Guessing or relying on patient assumptions can result in serious medication errors. Communication between pharmacists and prescribers ensures accurate, safe dispensing consistent with professional standards and patient safety protocols.

Q586. Answer: B

Explanation: In Category A, NCC MERP classifies situations with potential for error—conditions that could lead to a mistake if uncorrected. No actual error occurred. This proactive identification helps prevent future harm through corrective measures. Categories B–I represent increasing severity, from intercepted errors to those causing patient death. Recognizing Category A risks strengthens preventive safety culture.

Q587. Answer: B

Explanation: Patient safety is a shared responsibility. Technicians should confidentially report unsafe practices to a supervisor or pharmacist. Addressing potential breaches prevents harm and reinforces safety culture. Public confrontation risks conflict and violates professionalism, while inaction enables ongoing risk. Reporting ensures proper investigation and system-level corrective measures within a just, non-punitive framework.

Q588. Answer: A

Explanation: Proper handwashing with antimicrobial soap and warm water for at least 30 seconds removes microorganisms before donning gloves or entering cleanrooms. This is the foundation of aseptic compounding under USP <797>. Gloves and alcohol alone cannot replace mechanical washing. Touching supplies before washing risks contamination of sterile environments and compounded products.

Q589. Answer: B

Explanation: Any sterile item that falls on the floor or touches unclean surfaces is considered contaminated and must be discarded immediately. Alcohol wiping cannot restore sterility. USP <797> requires maintaining product integrity and replacing compromised items. Using contaminated materials risks patient infection or product recall. Safe handling protects both sterility and quality assurance.

Q590. Answer: A

Explanation: Misinterpreting unclear abbreviations or handwriting represents a communication error, one of the most common medication error sources. It occurs when verbal or written orders are misunderstood or ambiguous. Using standardized terminology and e-prescriptions reduces such risks. The other options are storage, environmental, or mechanical errors, not directly tied to communication failures.

Q591. Answer: C

Explanation: The United States Pharmacopeia (USP) establishes compounding and safety standards: <795> for nonsterile, <797> for sterile, and <800> for hazardous drug handling. These enforce consistency and protect patients and staff. The FDA enforces drug quality at the manufacturing level, while ISMP and CDC focus on medication safety and infection control, respectively.

Q592. Answer: B

Explanation: Independent double verification ensures accurate compounding calculations. Each technician or pharmacist should check drug concentrations, conversions, and volumes independently to catch potential arithmetic or unit errors. Estimation or mental shortcuts can cause dangerous overdoses or underdoses. Implementing calculator use and written verification supports precise preparation, fulfilling USP and CQI requirements.

Q593. Answer: A

Explanation: Using two unique identifiers—such as the patient's full name and date of birth—ensures accurate medication matching and prevents wrong-patient errors. Visual recognition or address verification alone can result in misidentification. This practice aligns with Joint Commission National Patient Safety Goals, emphasizing standardized procedures for verification before dispensing or administering medications.

Q594. Answer: A

Explanation: Controlled substances must be accurately documented at every handling stage—from receipt to dispensing to destruction—to maintain complete traceability. DEA regulations mandate detailed logs, witness verification, and daily reconciliation in many facilities. Skipping entries or sharing credentials violates federal law and undermines accountability. Thorough documentation ensures compliance and deters diversion.

Q595. Answer: D

Explanation: An error of omission occurs when a required medication is not administered or dispensed at all. This can lead to therapeutic failure or patient harm. Errors of commission, by contrast, involve incorrect actions such as wrong dose or patient. Documenting missed doses and investigating causes are vital to prevent recurrence in healthcare systems.

Q596. Answer: B

Explanation: Maintaining unobstructed airflow within the laminar flow hood ensures clean, particle-free air over compounding surfaces. Blocking airflow with supplies or hands disrupts sterile conditions, increasing contamination risk. Personal items and syringe reuse violate aseptic technique. Proper equipment placement and continual airflow monitoring are key USP <797> practices for environmental control.

Q597. Answer: B

Explanation: When storage temperature deviates from acceptable ranges, technicians must notify the pharmacist immediately and quarantine all affected drugs until stability verification. Temperature excursions can compromise potency, especially for biologics and vaccines. Ignoring or resetting without record violates QA policies. Documentation and corrective action ensure product integrity and regulatory compliance.

Q598. Answer: C

Explanation: Ongoing education and competency evaluations keep technicians updated on evolving safety, regulatory, and technological standards. It reinforces proper handling, labeling, and error-prevention techniques. Competency validation protects patients and supports accreditation. It's not just a formality—it's essential for sustaining professional development and maintaining high-quality pharmacy practice aligned with CQI initiatives.

Q599. Answer: C

Explanation: The FDA oversees the FAERS (FDA Adverse Event Reporting System), which collects post-marketing safety data on drugs and biologics. It helps identify new safety signals and guide regulatory actions. The CDC monitors public health and vaccines, the DEA controls controlled substances, and CMS focuses on healthcare reimbursement—not adverse drug reporting.

Q600. Answer: B

Explanation: A just culture balances accountability with a non-punitive environment that encourages open reporting of errors. Staff are held responsible for reckless behavior but not for system-based mistakes. This philosophy fosters transparency and continuous improvement. Punitive approaches discourage reporting, while tolerance for violations undermines safety. Just culture builds trust and drives sustainable quality assurance.

Made in United States
Orlando, FL
04 November 2026

90206052R00094